BACK

FROM

THE

BRINK

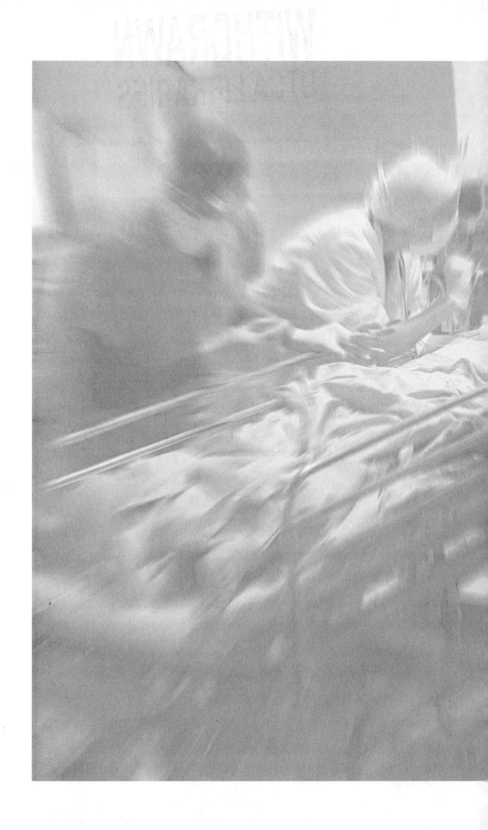

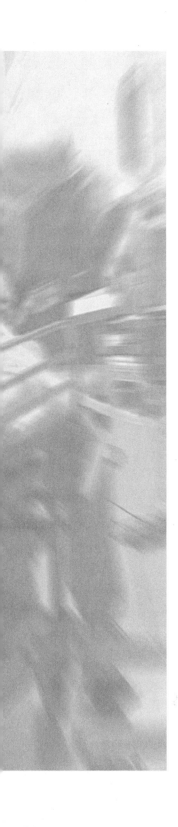

BACK

FROM

THE

BRINK

How Crises
Spur Doctors
to New Discoveries
about the Brain

Edward J. Sylvester

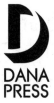

DANA
PRESS

New York | Washington, D.C.

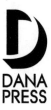

DANA
PRESS

Library of Congress Cataloging-in-Publication Data
Sylvester, Edward J.
  Back from the brink : how crises spur doctors to new discoveries about the brain / by Edward J. Sylvester.
    p. ; cm.
Includes bibliographical references and index.
  ISBN 0-9723830-4-2 (hardcover : alk. paper)
  1. Neurological emergencies. 2. Neurological emergencies—Case studies. 3. Brain--Localization of functions. 4. Mirski, Marek Alexander Z.--Contributions in neurological intensive care. 5. Mayer, Stephan A.--Contributions in neurological intensive care.
  [DNLM: 1. Mirski, Marek Alexander Z. 2. Mayer, Stephan A. 3. Johns Hopkins Hospital. 4. Columbia-Presbyterian Medical Center. 5. Brain Diseases--therapy. 6. Intensive Care Units. 7. Intensive Care. 8. Neurology--Biography. 9. Neurology--Case Report. WL 28 AM3 S985b 2003] I. Title.
  RC350.7.S97 2003
  616.8'0425--dc21

                                    2003010816

ISBN: 0-97238304-2

Cover/inside design by Jeff Potter/Potter Publishing Studio
Photo of Jeff and Gail Beck, courtesy of the Beck family
Medical illustrations Copyright 2003, Kathryn Born
Printed in the United States of America by Phoenix Color Corporation, Hagerstown, MD

THE DANA FOUNDATION
745 Fifth Avenue, Suite 900
New York, NY 10151

DANA PRESS
The Dana Center
900 15th Street NW
Washington, D.C. 20005

www.dana.org

FOR GINNY,

for always being there.

Contents

Author's Note

Back From The Brink is nonfiction, a true story—or rather, a series of true stories. Writing a work of fiction involves weaving together a complex web whose threads are of the author's imagination. Writing nonfiction can require weaving just as complex a web, but one whose threads trace to *sources*—real people who have shared their experiences, their observations, and their feelings for the author's record. Sometimes no one's permission is required for this, the underlying events being part of a public record. In this story, quite the opposite is the case. Very little of *Back From The Brink* occurs in anything like a public setting, and therefore hardly a word could have been written without the participants' permission—and more.

Because I have depicted real people dealing with major crises in their lives and with the physicians attempting to bring them back to health, the participants granted me access to private, often intensely personal details about themselves. And for the book to succeed in anything like "real time," they had to allow me to share the results at my discretion, without their having prior review of what I had written. Every patient and family member granted this request. Thus, all the episodes that follow are real; the relationships, events, quotations, and discussions are as accurate as I could render them. The result is journalism: there are no composite characters, invented scenes, or imagined dialogues. Without the extraordinary generosity of those you will read about, none of it would have been possible, and I am grateful to them beyond measure.

The identities of patients and their families are real as well, with one exception. The names of Michael Sanders and his wife, Marybeth Collins, are pseudonyms, at her request. Still, all that you will read of them and others I either witnessed or reconstructed from the accounts of those who were participants or witnesses. On the other hand, because the many people who figure prominently in the story are named, I decided not to give pseudonyms to patients encountered only in passing. Those patients are referred to simply, for example, as "George R____.

Most important, my discussing actual cases with doctors required patients to share their confidential medical information. Although not specifically noted as the story unfolds, each patient whose case is being discussed by his or her physician gave permission not only for me to use the material, but, to begin with, for the physician to speak with me about the case.

The ideas that would become this book developed over many years, and for most of those ideas I am indebted to many neuroscientists—Ph.D researchers as well as the clinician-investigators through whom the story develops. You will meet most of them. Many others, however, who were equally generous with their time in providing information or inspiration, do not appear in the text. Conversations with Arizona Health Sciences neurologist Scott Sherman, M.D. / Ph.D., beginning in 1998 got me thinking about the two very different "neuro" worlds that must be knit together by doctors like himself, who not only care for patients in hospital beds but who conduct vital research into the causes of the brain disorders they treat. The neurointensivists at the University of California San Francisco opened their two hospital units to me for several fascinating and important days, offering variations on the themes I had seen at Johns Hopkins and Columbia. And physicians such as Thomas Bleck of the University of Virginia, David Richman of the University of California Davis, and John Griffin, Donlin Long, and Henry Brem of Johns Hopkins provided valuable information and insight into the brain and into that other bewilderingly complex entity, the American medical center. In Munich, Gerhard Hamann, director of neurointensive care at the Neurologische Klinik, Ludwig-Maximilians-Universität, offered a wonderfully clear and concise picture of the differences and similarities between NICUs and their specialists in Germany and the United States, as well as a valuable look at his own state-of-the-art unit.

Finally, of course, no medical journalist can ever carry out his job without the support of those who support the physicians. At Johns Hopkins, Gloria McCoy and Pat Lamberti, the administrative specialists who keep the Division of Neurosciences Critical Care ticking, kept me connected and informed as well. At Columbia, Robert Kowalski and Shelley Peery, research assistants for the Neurological Intensive Care Unit, proved as invaluable resources for me as they are for their unit, as did administrative assistant Betty Politi.

The neurosciences comprise several professions whose members spend many years learning not only the extraordinarily difficult skills of their crafts but the equally difficult ways of speaking precisely about brain science. Attempting to describe and explain their work in ordinary language leaves any journalist open to error at every turn. Peter Raudzens, head of neuroanesthesia at Barrow Neurological Institute, read the manuscript to catch medical errors, misstatements, and especially the kinds of imprecision that can mislead readers. To him and to the other medical professionals who read the manuscript in advance of publication, I am deeply grateful. Naturally, the errors that managed to get through are mine alone.

This Author's Note, like most for works of nonfiction, is a catalog of my indebtedness to the real fountainheads of the story. Such sources cannot be repaid, but perhaps they can best be thanked by telling their stories well. I hope that I have done so. If I have succeeded, it has certainly not been through my efforts alone. Jane Nevins, my outstanding editor at Dana Press, believed in this book when it was a series of rough chapter sketches. She supported me at every turn over two years, and, by far most important, caught so much that needed work in each successive draft, yet never missed what was right, even when I did, and never wavered in her belief in the book that is, at last, in hand.

A U.S. Doctor's Progress

Medical Training Required For 3 M.D. Career Paths

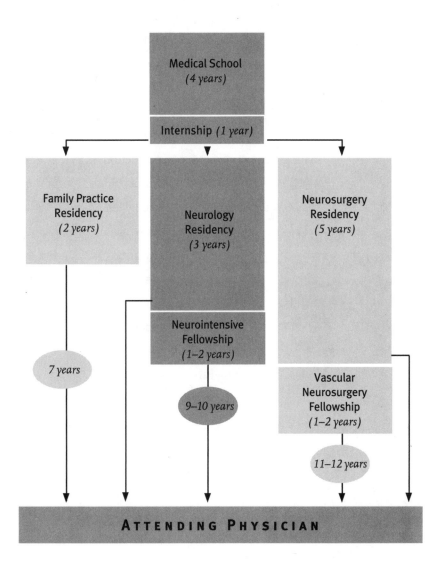

Grand Rounds

June 6, 2001

A WARM MARYLAND SUN broke the rim of sky as Dr. Marek Mirski headed from home, south of Baltimore, at his routine hour around dawn. But his destination was not usual. Normally he drove downtown, and his route might take him across the Orleans Street bridge, soaring above the rail yards to catch sight of the vast and growing complex of Johns Hopkins Hospital with the sun rising behind it. There he leads one of the world's top programs in training and directing specialists who treat brain-injured patients.

Today he drove to the Amtrak station, bound for Columbia's New York Presbyterian Hospital. The whole purpose of his trip was to deliver a message. He had been invited to give grand rounds in neurology, hosted by his Columbia counterpart, Dr. Stephan Mayer, and he would report from his upcoming journal article on results of a study with important implications for their field.

Marek would be introduced as "Mark," as he always pronounces it, and, taking the podium, he would deliver his findings in his usual unassuming manner. He is no preacher. An MIT graduate, M.D./Ph.D. from Washington University, and a brain doctor at one of the world's great academic medical centers, he would make his case to Columbia's physicians with hard evidence and little fanfare. Mayer could do grand rounds on terminal procedures and bring bursts of laughter from the crowd. Mirski would provide food for thought.

He also had little use for the bellicose imagery of "disease wars" or the military-style discipline and punishing training regimens of earlier generations of medical leaders, but he set himself the same goals with the same determination. So removed was his easygoing manner from the gung-ho abrasiveness of the typical TV doctor that he was once upbraided by a patient's wife because she mistook his quietly authoritative manner for inattention. She later admitted she was expecting the barked orders and shouted observations she had witnessed over her TV-viewing years. It wasn't as though Mirski had never seen that kind of behavior in the flesh, but to him it was unprofessional. Professional meant in control, steady, confident, yet ever-watchful for the unexpected. It was also clear that his style met with the approval of his superiors.

If you were brought into his Neurological Intensive Care Unit, that meant your life was threatened by injury or disease to your brain. Mirski and his team would get you out alive, if they could find a way, whether tried-and-true or discovered in a desperate moment. Any intensive care unit is about rescues, some heroic, all difficult. Neuro tells that the rescues must be made in the strangest and most complex terrain so far

known in the universe: the human brain. Groundbreaking discoveries
in the news about how the brain functions and why it fails, and all the
theories, studies, and pie-in-the-sky hopes about what it takes to heal
dying brains, come hurtling to earth right here in the Neuro ICU. You
can see them work or not.

I would spend this summer of 2001 and parts of the next two years
in Mirski's Neuro ICU at Johns Hopkins Hospital, in an arcane world that
grew slowly familiar, round by round. I got there by choice, working out
one of those obsessions that grip you and won't let go, which invariably take
root as a question too big to get your mind around. Such as: how does the
brain work? For me as a science writer, insights come in the form of stories, so there was no better place to look than where some of the smartest
and most skilled people are not only grappling with the question but actually assembling pieces of answers.

The Neuro ICU is the world of the neurointensivist, as Mirski, Mayer,
and the tiny cadre they train are called. Some neurointensivists begin as
neurologists passionate to take action in the fight to save lives, not content
to diagnose and back away. Some are neuroanesthesiologists whose op-
erating-room training gave them expertise with the physical tools of keeping the brain-injured alive, driven to develop their skills beyond the OR doors
by applying the rescue skills of the neurosurgical team to the critical healing process that follows. Some, like Mirski, trained as both neurologists
and anesthesiologists.

In the tough medical world of the new century, neurointensivists aim
to establish themselves as the first-line rescuers in the brain, the chiefs
of the specialized neurological ICUs springing up in medical centers
around the world. They were my guides into the workings of the brain
and the myriad threats to it that teach as much as do the tools of rescue.
Like emergency physicians, they are crisis managers. Watching them suc-

ceed and fail revealed more of the inner workings of the brain than I had believed one could witness.

The brain as object looms over this specialized world, yet the deeper one delves, the odder it seems to call the brain an object. The reality of the brain as it comes ever-clearer at higher and higher resolution, at some deep point seems to give way to another reality altogether. Like the physical world in the realm of the quark, somewhere on the downward brain journey, a very important "it" vanishes from the screen. You can weigh the brain at autopsy—about three pounds of tissue—and hold it. It feels rubbery, but that's because of preservative. In the brain's living years, even scaffolded by support cells, the neuronal filigree would collapse without its tough enclosing membranes.

Turn it all ways, like Yorick's skull. Behold the person, minus only the person. That's the strangeness. The brain represents the boundary of objective reality. It forms out of the same genetic program that fits together the same molecules that build our viscera and skeletons. Yet in the most important sense, the brain finally assembles itself, bootstrapping hundreds of billions of its cells into the right positions, where they somehow lure each other into making the right trillions of connections—some before birth, most in response to living, as learning. Strange. Just think. Remember. Wonder. How does wonder, or any of the rest, emerge out of cells? Yet kill the cells, and all the rest goes away, in part or in whole.

More than in Baltimore—or New York or any other stop on a two-year journey—this story takes place in the brain, and the Neuro ICU is its planetary space, the place of pioneering efforts to heal and restore it and to extend its life.

All critical-care physicians, like emergency room doctors, thrive on pressure, excitement, hands-on involvement in patient care and rescue. Yet for all their expertise, Mirski says, most general critical-care specialists will not venture into the land of the brain. Neurologists, by contrast, are stereotyped by other physicians as "pipe smokers"—reflective, cerebral, dispassionate. Masters of the one organ most others will not deal with, yet above the fray.

It's hard to imagine two neurologists who are more different from this stereotype than Marek Mirski and Stephan Mayer, yet the sharp contrasts between their own personalities illustrate the enormous range of physicians drawn to this medical frontier.

Mirski's manner *is* reflective and cerebral, and his cool gives the appearance of detachment, even in the middle of the worst of catastrophes he puts his hands to daily—in fact, especially at such moments. Nothing is more antithetical to the approach he practices and teaches than stridency, impatience, or loss of personal control. But he is never aloof.

Now take Mayer, his host. He loves to joke, to solve problems on his feet, to give and take with his team on rounds, in repartée. On our first meeting, a year earlier, Mayer had cited an old saw of medicine: "There are only two things a neurologist needs to know: Diagnose and, 'Adios!'" You can hear the drum rap. "Guys with great questions and no answers"—a rim shot—"who know everything and do nothing." But said above a cacophony of monitors and conversation, as still other monitors entered the shrill music of medical emergency with whistles, bells, or strange, minor chords of alerts. The tired adages were only good for a joke here.

Although most of this story takes place at Johns Hopkins, Mayer's Columbia offered a harrowing look at two lives that brought into sharp focus some of the most elusive qualities of personality. They had nothing in common except a Long Island town and their passage through his NICU, but they emerged in a single story, a parable of the brain's abilities and limitations.

On that earlier summer morning when we had first met, Mayer's powers to heal and to decide were tested twice within an hour. First, he made a decision to try to rescue a man so near death many physicians would have declared him hopeless; and then a second decision, to let a young woman slip into death, as she had expressly wished, by turning off her respirator rather than save her for the life-in-death known as a persistent vegetative state. But turning off a respirator is not passive. The new world of neuro rescue has brought us to the hardest ethical questions of medical practice. Mayer firmly believed that if he turned off the young woman's respirator, she would die. He did so, and she did. But Mayer would offer the larger world of neurointensive care more than the two stories that will serve here as counterpoint. He also would play a major role in organizing the diverse neurointensivists into a new medical association, the Neurocritical Care Society.

As the train rolled through the coastal hills of the Chesapeake watershed and into the flat of Delaware, then crossed the river into southern New Jersey, Mirski was no more aware of the changing terrain than he was of the pathways of his thoughts as he ruminated over the fields of data. The data formed the foundation of his message, and he had sliced and diced it countless times to reassure himself there was no weak spot in the foundation—or at least, none that he had not already seen. But obsession with numbers and measurement is hardly limited to science. We are awash in data. We, or specialist members of our professional teams, calculate correlations between data sets for PowerPoint presentations, like shamans brooding over entrails, before making on-screen pronouncements. Knowledge is power, and in our world knowledge is built out of observed fact, increasingly represented by numbers.

The numbers Mirski would present, he believed and hoped, represented enormous medical power in years to come.

Arriving at New York's Penn Station, he took the subway to 168 Street, then walked west toward the Hudson River, to Columbia's Millstein Building. At 10 a.m., about a hundred physicians gathered for grand rounds in the main auditorium overlooking the river and the Palisades.

In making daily hospital rounds, small groups of physicians move from patient to patient, going over treatment notes, generalizing from this case to others, observing, contrasting, prescribing. Grand rounds meetings bring together an entire department, with invitations to others to join in, usually in such an auditorium. They range from summations of recent cases with a common theme—as the *grand* might imply—to more formal presentations of clinical data supporting a particular protocol, the sort of presentation offered in science conferences. Mirski's would be the latter.

He steps to the podium, the room quiets, and he begins. Ready for this? If you're like me, probably not. Mirski's is a scientific message, and for most of us there are two big problems with scientific messages. First, they are way too *short*. Too much is packed into sentences of a few words, each word carrying an enormous freight of information and force of meaning. Therefore years of training are needed—intellectual weight training—to heft and turn them with knowing ease. Second, the messages are almost invariably nested in beds of numbers. For the uninitiated, hearing the data chanted out—assertion, question, response—is like beholding the ritual of an alien religion, incomprehensible even in our native tongue. Mirski's message was for the initiated, so although his conclusions and comments were in plain enough English, all the supporting evidence was not. There's no record of the talk, but here is a key point from the in-press journal article it was based on, in which he refers more formally to the Neuro Sciences Intensive Care Unit:

"Primary neurosurgical populations admitted to the NSICU during FY 1997 included patients with postoperative craniotomies with and without intracranial hemorrhage (A-DRGs 001 and 002) ..." So far, okay. Then, "Adjusting for severity of illness, patients treated in the NSICU on average spent 4.5 ± 0.4 (SEM) days in the ICU after craniotomy if they had a hemorrhage (A-DRG 001; HBSI ICU reference benchmark, 6.0 ± 0.5 days) and 1.8 ± 0.2 days if there was no hemorrhage (A-DRG 002; benchmark 2.9 ± 0.2 days)."

Enough! Since the message concerns life and death, it's worth the effort to unpack it.

Say your brain is dying, and the ambulance speeding you to rescue comes to a fork in the road. Each path leads to a critical care unit where you will get close scrutiny and intense support from equally fine doctors. There is only one variable. At one unit, you will be met by your own doctor, who will summon experts who, hopefully, will have the power to save you, body and mind. At the other, you will be met by a neurointensivist who will take charge of your care, superseding not only your own doctor but all others called to the scene as consultants, however able and experienced they might be.

Mirski's message: at the NICU run by a trained neurointensivist, you have a better chance of living. Next, you have a better chance of leaving the ICU sooner. And finally, leaving, the chances are better that the whole course of treatment will cost less.

An easy choice? Maybe, but let's not jump to that conclusion.

Did Mirski really study all the outcomes in the dozens of neuro and general ICUs in America, compiling the data from each, carefully mining that mountain and drilling out relevant numbers, over enough years to achieve "statistically significant results"? That would have taken a decade or more, even if he could have gotten all the data. He had studied one midsize Neuro Science Intensive Care Unit that he had set up and run in Hawaii, and he had looked at the patient recoveries outlined above for two separate years—one before it had become specialized for neurointensive care and one during his administration. The same doctors treated the same categories of injury and illness in one state's population using the same tools—but under a different aegis. Result: different outcomes. Mirski's implicit premise this morning is that this world he holds up for inspection is a microcosm, that he has painstakingly distilled a pure essence from the inscrutable larger world. Doing so, after all, is a major purpose of the tortuous process of data analysis: to generalize from a manageable handful of data to a mass we may not even gauge. This is a key part of science. He challenges his supporters to join him in the knowledge-mining venture, as he will challenge doubters and disbelievers, as smart and dedicated as he is, to come up with data that prove him wrong.

After the applause as his talk concludes, questions and challenges are posed and addressed, and grand rounds draws to a close.

SO THE BATTLE IS ALWAYS JOINED, but it would hardly be of interest to us if it were all a numbers war, destined to remain obscure to all but a few. But look at where Mirski and Mayer find themselves—not literally, having post-rounds lunch in a neighborhood Dominican restaurant, but figuratively, the critical context of their conversation.

Here in the early twenty-first century, medicine in the United States dances on the edge of a strange chaos. Hospitals are closing at an unprecedented rate, and many of those that stay in business are eliminating whole wings full of beds—often quietly, aiming to get under the public radar, because such closings represent failure of a huge investment. Doctors who have trained for half their lives quit in their prime, in disgust over the restrictions of managed care or unable to pay rocketing malpractice premiums, and that represents an even greater loss of both capital and personal investment. That notwithstanding, without some form of managed care the system would be bankrupt, and doctors know it. As serious as these crises are, they are just markers for the turmoil that lies beneath.

Yet never has such a rush of discoveries poured down every pathway to dazzle heart and mind. Some are the outgrowth of the most careful, painstaking science, representing the accretions of quiet efforts by investigators who brave years of mind-numbing tedium without going numb, like Antarctic explorers. Other achievements arrive serendipitously, entirely unexpected. Breakthroughs forecast decades from now seem to fall in our laps.

So here is a paradox: with the overall number of patients in U.S. hospitals plummeting, more patients than ever are being admitted to ICUs, and those admitted are sicker than they used to be. Advances across the realms of medical treatment mean that patients who once were simply cared for till they died now emerge very much alive. In the Neuro ICU, they come from neurosurgery and interventional radiology to join sufferers of formerly deadly hemorrhages and other strokes, and once-mysterious ailments like Guillain-Barré syndrome, on a long, expensive road to recovery. Who is running all these intensive care units? Their directors come from a spectrum of specialties, though general intensivists have been recognized subspecialists in internal medicine for many years. Some ICU directors are simply internists with no further specialization, some are anesthesiologists, others are surgeons. Put neuro in front of ICU, and the same range of directors is found.

Now a powerful group pushing for medical reform was demanding that trained intensivists run all intensive care units. The Leapfrog Group comprises Fortune 500 companies and others who are the payers of medical insurance. In the first Leapfrog report, the industrialists suggested they would push to no longer pay for any other model of intensive care: intensive care units, they said, must be run by intensivists.

For Mirski, this was the perfect moment for the kind of evidence about neurointensivists he had presented at grand rounds and would soon be publishing. The Leapfrog report suggested that their little-known subspecialty might become ubiquitous, if they could train enough people and prove the demand. The problem is that *intensivist* does not necessarily mean *neurointensivist*. The critical care subspecialty for brain treatment had never been formally recognized. Overcoming that hurdle was Mirski's and Mayer's goal. Those who completed Johns Hopkins's two-year fellowship to be certified neurointensivists were already in such demand that Mirski had trouble keeping them until they became seasoned enough to run their own Neuro ICUs, and Mayer had had to run his own unit single-handedly until recently. Now the numbers of demand had to be brought down to concrete and steel, "patient-hours" translated into numbers of beds for the patients, square feet of space for the beds.

Both Johns Hopkins and Columbia were planning major expansions of their Neuro ICUs, and both neurointensive training programs were begun at the same time, by pioneers in the field. But the differences between the units were at least as great as the similarities, and they showed the breadth of realities into which a single idea had evolved in just 20 years.

Mayer ran the Neuro ICU here and was responsible for every patient in it, but it was a shared responsibility. Columbia's is an "open" unit, meaning that neurosurgeons and others manage their own NICU patients. The major force in the creation of the Neuro ICU as a specialty unit was neurosurgery, and neurosurgeons still dominate the units in many if not most American hospitals.

Johns Hopkins's, by contrast, is a "closed" unit, and this is no small distinction when you are the patient being wheeled from neurosurgery and you ask, "Who is my doctor?" At Johns Hopkins, the answer is the neurointensivist in charge of the NICU, regardless of who your neurosurgeon or admitting physician was.

Most units are more like Columbia's, by necessity if not choice. Because the supply of neurointensivists cannot keep up with demand, from a nationwide perspective, sharing responsibility for patient care is a must. But Johns Hopkins offers the purest example of what a neurointensivist does and aims to do, which is to manage the whole patient, even though he or she was admitted for neurological problems. More of these specialists have trained at Hopkins than anywhere else in America, and, by far, more of those now running programs were trained there under Daniel Hanley than under any other mentor. Hanley founded Johns Hopkins's NICU, ran it for some 15 years, and is one of four doctors everyone cites as the fathers of the concept.

THE COLUMBIA ARCHITECT'S BLUEPRINTS were unrolled across a conference table outside Mayer's windowless eighth-floor office, pulled from their shelf as Mirski and Mayer returned from lunch, and we huddled to see what would emerge. As they go over the expansion, I see the story's Neuro ICU taking shape in the blue-line drawing before us. It's a measure of the newness of these specialized units that even their names have variations as you move from hospital to hospital. At Columbia, it's the Neurointensive Care Unit. At Johns Hopkins, The Neuroscience Critical Care Unit, at others the Neuro Sciences Critical Care Unit; each, of course, breeds its own alphabet soup of an acronym.

But from the beginning, and in conversational shorthand everywhere, NICU is the common term. So it will be here, fixed and concrete as the unit itself will become in the pages ahead as people are added and subtracted. People are the vital force. On this June day, they have just returned from lunch, to offices or college classrooms, or to resume household chores or go shopping for dinner. Not all of them will be alive next June.

Drug abuse got Jay Lokeman at 34, on the streets of Baltimore, though the immediate cause of his being brought in was the relentless storm of seizures in the brain called *status epilepticus*. The struggling sibling in a family of intensely competitive high achievers, he would soon be surrounded by family members for as many hours in the day as rules allowed, all praying he would survive and emerge as the man he could be.

Then there are those two Long Island patients, so clearly paired in my mind though they've never met, who passed through the Columbia NICU exactly four years apart. Gail Beck, 32, had no accident, no symptoms, no history—none of those subtle warning signs that might be missed ahead of time but that stand out glaringly afterward. From healthy mother of two in Huntington Station, Long Island, in a flash she became a comatose Columbia patient on a downward spiral. Michael Sanders, 45, went out for cigarettes in Massapequa, Long Island, on Father's Day, dropped like a stone at a gas station cashier's window, and was lucky enough to be seen by a licensed practical nurse filling up at the next island. Next seen, he lay in a profound coma from which his neurointensivist and his wife vowed to bring him back.

Vassar junior Jennie Ray, just turned 21, came home to north Baltimore for the summer. She passed out from an undiscovered arteriovenous malformation and now writhed in agony in the Johns Hopkins Neuro ICU. Donna Soja, 28, had been in the same bed a day earlier after a helicopter flight from Delaware, and she had chatted with the nurses and anesthesiologist about their kids as she was wheeled in to neurosurgery. A day after Jennie came in, Rita Serianni, 56, lay next to her, felled by a stroke as she cleaned up for the evening in her Columbia, Maryland, kitchen.

Time is brain, stroke specialists say. Jack Apple, 61, clutched his head and groaned in pain, and his wife, Ellen, soon set out on a nightmare trip through Baltimore streets closed by construction zones, desperate to get him to the emergency room. But a far worse trip was to come. Sooner or later, Jack Apple would recover or die—or worse, enter the perpetual gray zone of vegetative existence.

The NICU is at once an island of peace, a clean well-lighted place, and a harbinger of dread, the next-to-last place you ever hope to be. The last place, of course, is in the situation that brought you through these doors. But if that is already a given, this is where you want to be taken, where you will most likely be rescued. Hose by joint it was designed that way. Like most medical innovations, the NICU was hammered out of the wreckage of failed responses to brain trauma by a very small number of doctors, beginning only two decades ago. And like so many great human creations, it was born out of necessity but built using all the determination, intellect, and stamina its founders could muster. It remains, as you will see, a monument to clashing wills, opposing visions, and what the devil or chance can wreak on the stage of the human brain.

The best time to look in is always at night, when it's quiet. No monitors shriek or hum inane tunes to get your attention. A soft bell tone will rivet the nurse's eye to the appropriate monitor at her station just outside her patients' doors. When ambulances arrive at night, you can hear the sirens coming for blocks, their wails alternately blocked and amplified by the building. But when the sirens stop, the next sound you wait for is soft: a dulcet-toned, usually female computer voice calling the trauma team to the emergency room. And if required, the evening's last stop might be here in the NICU—"the unit," to its nurses and physicians.

Such units usually are horseshoe-shaped, with patient rooms lining the outer walls on three sides. That leaves the center of the horseshoe for mission control—the nurses' desk with phones, computers hardwired to the hospital's mainframe, paper records.

Morning and evening, the white-coated team rounds the outer rim in a shifting cluster, usually with a cart between them carrying patient charts, and they will spend anywhere from 10 to 20 minutes, sometimes longer, going over each patient's status. The team includes an attending neurointensivist and fellow, joined by specialists called in for consults, and residents in neurology and neurosurgery, plus neurosurgeons discussing their own patients, then leaving, and, at Johns Hopkins, the NICU nurses.

A unique touch at one NICU is worth mentioning. Someone at Arizona Medical Center in Tucson noticed that patients regaining consciousness were staring up at the glossy light panels, suddenly confronted by their own reflections. Some were terrified at this first sight of themselves transformed, swathed in bandages, black-eyed and bloodied. So now the ceiling light panel of each patient's room depicts a glorious scene of wilderness terrain, maybe red rock from the Grand Canyon or Monument Valley, or skyscraping mountains, cheerful sunny meadows or green glens bubbling water. Better this postcard vision at first light.

BACK IN THE REAL WORLD, Marek Mirski completed his circle, reversing course for Penn Station and walking in his door in suburban Baltimore's Severna Park before sundown, just as Stephan Mayer would be reaching the brownstone downtown from Columbia he had left that morning. Round and round they go—a phrase that can have opposite connotations. Going in circles, running the rat race—going nowhere. Or circling steadily in or out, now up, now down like a gyrfalcon, each circle marking a new power of resolution, or articulation, or achievement. Looked at this close, there's no telling which meaning, eventually, will mark today.

CHAPTER 1

Wreckers Ball

June 30, 2001

STANDING ON THE highest roof in the Johns Hopkins Hospital complex, you are at one of the finest vantage points in Baltimore, the great port and crossroads that invested the new United States with its first network of westward expansion, wagon roads through the Cumberland Gap. Two centuries later medicine is the city's major commerce, and this is its hub. Johns Hopkins is the largest employer in Baltimore, and the largest, other than government, in the entire state of Maryland.

The view takes in the whole city and its vast in-sweep of Chesapeake Bay. The Inner Harbor glitters to the south and west, and although it's too far away to see the tourists thronging its shops and pathways, there's no better place than this roof to watch the fireworks that will be shot off for their entertainment next week on the Fourth of July.

It was Dr. Daniel Hanley who commended the view as the best in the city. No matter how long you lived here, he said, "You might never know how beautiful Baltimore is if you had never seen it from that vantage." He had said it by way of analogy, to illustrate a very different idea. No matter how well you might come to know the brain and its destroyers, however intimately in thousands of cases, successes and failures stretching over decades, in key ways you would only understand its complexity by getting above it—that is, as an epidemiologist would. Look out over the vast rolling hills of data, the topology of research amassed over decades, throughout the world, and see the patterns. Hanley has now turned his career toward that seeing. Probably no perspective better reflects the Johns Hopkins idea of medicine as I would come to see it and hear it explained, yet Hanley has always regarded himself as something of an outsider to the Hopkins way, a survivor on one of the most competitive pieces of medical turf in the world, by dint of medical skill, pluck, and shrewdness. He has reached an apex not everyone achieves, full professorship, with an endowed chair, at that.

Two decades ago, Hanley and nurse manager Ski Lower created the Neuro ICU eight floors below us; more than that, they pioneered the idea of a neurointensivist team of physicians and nurses to manage it. Two decades is brief in the life of a hospital or a city. Down below, to the west of the Adolf Meyer building that houses the NICU, sits the Phipps Psychiatric Clinic, built in 1906 as one of Hopkins's early buildings, in whose garden a visiting John Steinbeck supposedly wrote during one summer in the thirties. In 1938, one of the most famous neurosurgeons of all time, Walter Dandy, operated on one of America's most famous writers, Thomas Wolfe, suspecting that the author had tuberculosis of the brain and hoping it might be treatable. To his dismay, Dandy found Wolfe's brain covered in tubercles and could do nothing but close. Wolfe died here that year, on September 15. Among his lesser known achievements, Dandy pioneered the concept of an intensive care unit to continue the close monitoring of critically ill patients leaving the operating room. Across the street is Church Home and Hospital, where Edgar Allan Poe died on October 7, 1849, of what may have been rabies inflaming his brain. But two decades is an age in modern medicine, marking an era just ended, whose founding lies at the heart of this story.

Most of the twentieth century had passed when, in 1982, Hopkins Neurosurgery chief Donlin Long tapped a young Daniel F. Hanley Jr. to create a subspecialty for the intensive care of brain-injured patients. His model would be a course started by Allan Ropper at Massachusetts General Hospital. At that time, there was neither a neurointensivist nor a place for one to work, just that idea. Recruitment was mostly by word of mouth, the lure for most fellows embodied in one word: *action*. Michael Diringer, one of Hanley's first hires, is a prototype. He remembers casting about for a specialty that would combine his interest in the brain and its communicating molecules—its pharmacology—with hands-on action. He could not bear the idea of spending his days talking in a clinic, so he had abandoned a residency in psychiatry. Ropper had the neurointensivist course to offer him but, at the time, no fellowship money for training, Diringer recalls, so he recommended Johns Hopkins. He and Jeffrey Kirsch arrived together, following Robert Hansen and Mark Feldman, and, under Hanley as neurologist and Cecil Borel as anesthesiologist, they became Johns Hopkins's first graduated neurointensivists.

Like many of Hanley's trainees, Diringer now runs a highly regarded Neuro ICU and training program, at Washington University in St. Louis.

There, in turn, he trained one of this year's two fellows, Diana Greene-Chandos, as a neurologist.

Hanley, just starting out in 1982, has moved on in new directions with new vigor, at that middle age when many physicians are just assuming directorships and as many others are planning retirement. He was that young at the founding. The NICU is moving on as well, having evolved beyond one person's and one generation's vision. Hanley and the NICU are, in a real sense, divorced. Amicably perhaps, but divorced.

D UE   WEST   OF   M EYER   are the towers of downtown, attractively modern but indistinguishable from almost any other city's high-rise cluster. Northward lie the leafy, comfortable neighborhoods surrounding and extending north from Johns Hopkins University's main campus in Homewood. Finally, turning east, you can see Bayview Medical Center towering a few miles distant, part of the Hopkins medical complex that will offer a major challenge to Marek Mirski and the neurointensivist team in just a few days.

But let's not ignore the immediate on this gorgeous summer Saturday, the sprawling neighborhoods of east and central Baltimore, most of them desperately poor, some neat and working class. The whole is as intensely urban as cities get in their mix of apartment buildings, projects and double- and triple-decker homes and rentals. Johns Hopkins, meanwhile, is on the growth edge of a booming, international industry—medical care. And as a result of that boom, everywhere in the gritty blocks surrounding us, wrecking balls destroy the old row houses and factories, and construction crews send up new towers and pavilions of Johns Hopkins Hospital, with more to come. Church Home and Hospital was traded to Johns Hopkins by the city for other land, and the wrecking cranes are at work over there, too.

Hopkins flies its banners before the entire world, drawing patients from every country, their families often staying at special rates at pricey Inner Harbor hotels. It's a United Nations-like assemblage, with both the treated and those treating them growing in number and diversity each year. Conversely, this hospital-city that is also a major corporation with multinational footprint may one day offer the hands of a Baltimore neurosurgeon, robotically, to a patient half a world away—perhaps at the up-and-running Johns Hopkins/Singapore.

Much of this growth, at the expense of housing, has caused friction with neighbors, especially among minority groups whose poorer members are least able to pick up and hunt for new apartments. Clashes of urban universities and medical centers with their neighborhoods are not uncommon, nor are they ignored here. But they are signs of the times in medicine, and these are times of stark contrasts.

Below us, side-by-side with world potentates of government and business are many patients who make it to the emergency room on their last legs, either without insurance or having been denied coverage by their insurance companies. That leaves the hospital to cover the cost of caring for them by charging payers $6 for an aspirin; the anesthesia drug fentanyl was billed at nearly its exorbitant street price as "gentleman's heroin" until a generic became available in operating rooms. All this turmoil is part of the greatest period of discovery about the human body and brain ever, with nothing but the promise of more to come. Still, none of it distinguishes Johns Hopkins from half a dozen other major American medical centers, which collectively are the paradigm emulated by the more numerous hospitals in the next tier of regional medical centers.

In one arena, however, Johns Hopkins Medical Institutions stands as epitome, champ. This is the quintessential American medical-research complex. Its 1,810 full-time faculty investigators lead in defining evidence-based medicine, and the faculty promotion policies of Johns Hopkins Medicine could be a model for any Research Level I American university. No other institution comes close to garnering the $408 million in sponsored-research grants, mostly from the National Institutes of Health, that will flow to Johns Hopkins this year. Of that, $277.5 million will go for research on people in 2,400 separate studies going on at this moment.

In a few days, *U.S. News & World Report* will rank Johns Hopkins the best of the best hospitals in America for 2001, for the eleventh straight year, a ranking determined largely by peer evaluations. Surely in terms of leadership in finding answers—new cures, new drugs, new protocols—this is *the* place, everyone at Hopkins will agree as they celebrate the selection. Yet some will wryly turn the accolade into a question. Given its recognized superiority in patient care, why doesn't the hospital rank clinical service more highly when evaluating physicians for promotion, or in evaluating the department heads who mentor them? Research and publication rank well ahead of clinical service in those bottom-line evaluations. Of course, patient care is the top priority of every physician *on service* in every operating room and at every bedside. But in evaluating physicians, research and publication are tops. Beneath our feet, science rules.

That's the wide-angle view, the world of dollars and percentages. Incidences. Odds ratios. Correlations. Where science rules, laws are written in numbers, dotted with Greek. At eye level, where we live, the numbers jump, dance, run out of order, collide, fall over. More often than not, in the common idiom, it's all Greek.

Down below, for example, a collision of these worlds is in progress.

Somewhere in the streets, Jay Lokeman has scored a round of cocaine or heroin and maybe at this moment he is enjoying the intense, short-lived pleasure. At 34, he has known lots of such moments, but little peace. His family, who love him wholly and soon will prove it, lay the blame for that turmoil right at his feet. They personify tough love, and they will prove that too. His mother, Ardelia, whom he has promised countless times that he would stay clean, is a leader in Ebenezer Baptist Church, one of Baltimore's oldest, where her grandmother was a charter member. Jay is Ardelia's son with her second husband, James Sr. His siblings, the Reids, each represent a kind of success that can be won only by discipline, hard work and competitive drive. Vernon, the eldest at 47, is a fund manager for a major investment house. Cathy is a Red Cross executive. Joey is a Harvard-educated business lawyer. Where, exactly, does the youngest fit in?

Vernon admits he knew little of his younger brother, more than a decade his junior, who was just growing up when Vernon was a young adult. What was he like? "He's my mother's nicest kid," Vernon says simply. A superb athlete, gifted in tennis and swimming, not much interested in study, as a young man Jay had easily gotten jobs as a coach, lifeguard or athletic trainer. A man of easy grace and great charm to whom friends, and girlfriends, came easily. Maybe he had too much charm, and maybe all things came too easily.

No matter now. Soon Jay will be consumed with terror. Until recently he had been off drugs for months, working steadily at his job in collections for a mortgage company, doing the math, paying the rent. He had been clean since the wake-up call he'd gotten in March, the last time he went "rippin' and runnin'," going from the occasional recreational drug use into overdrive, topping out in the paranoia that sent him racing headlong into the streets. Then, he had run into the path of a car, reflexively stuck out his arms, and been flung over the hood. He spent weeks in the hospital and more months with his arms stuck out before him in casts, but he'd stayed clean. Until it began again. Now he is rushing headlong from his apartment in north Baltimore, in full flight, desperate to get to the shelter of his father's apartment in a retirement home downtown. His father could usually calm him down, and he could do chores for his father. Jay Sr. had been living there for many years because diabetes had compounded an unusual, apparently inherited tendency toward extremely low blood pressure that had forced amputation of both legs while he was still fairly young.

Much as Jay wants to quit, his brain screams for a fix, a few billion neurons all signaling *want.* Jay's problem is all chemical in origin, *and* it is all in his head. It consumes his imagination and drains his spirit, and it is real as rain.

Eat your favorite food when you are famished and you will feel intense pleasure, chemically induced. Serotonin and other molecules of your brain's own chemical stores, most assembled on-site from building blocks, will flood centers that evolved over millions of years for only one purpose, and that purpose is *to reward good behavior.* Eating leads to survival, so it is very good behavior. But in the for-keeps game of evolution, no behavior is better than that which leads to the survival and sowing of your genes, which is immortality. Make love, and even more of the chemicals of joy and pleasure flood those brain centers, all the more intensely. In the game of evolution, reproducing trumps even your own survival as worthy of the reward of feeling pleasure.

But if you do drugs, you can sometimes get all those rewards—food and sex distilled into a hypodermic shot—for doing absolutely nothing toward your or anyone's survival. The drugs mimic your brain's chemicals and often beat them at bringing pleasure. Evolution's gold is hijacked. You can destroy yourself, your genes, your mate, your offspring, and you can feel ecstatic while doing it—just don't stop. Jay has no wife, no children, and he has never hurt anyone but himself; he wants to stop. He runs the miles to see his father at his retirement home downtown. He truly wants to quit.

What happened next? There are too many versions and their edges don't match, maybe an analog for what's going on now in Jay's brain. He had a seizure, that much seems plain. Each of the hundred billion cells in his brain had been firing in its prescribed frequency, according to its type and location, from a few times a second at the fastest to a few times a minute or less, the firing of one leading to the firing of others in patterns too intricate to describe, like a concert of fireflies that light and frogs that sing perfect harmonies across the vast meadows of the cerebral cortex. Such patterns give rise to Jay himself, as they give rise to you and me, fireflies, frogs, all creatures with a brain.

Because of the drugs, infection, exhaustion, or the dissonance brought on by all of them, perhaps even because of the craving brought on by his efforts to stay clean, one loop of brain cells went on a firing binge, its steady thrum screaming out of control. Now the seizure loop kindled other circuits. But how did he come to be fighting with cops? They were sent to intercept a black male possibly on drugs raging in the parking lot of a downtown apartment building.

WHILE ALL THIS IS GOING ON in the streets below, seven floors up in Johns Hopkins Hospital, the Neuro ICU rattles and clatters with movers, making way for expansion. On Monday, the workers' drill drivers, crow bars and saws will tear out the Neuro Progressive Care Unit— a step-down between the Neuro ICU and those general hospital units that are collectively known as "the floor," as in "This patient is well enough to go to the floor today." Once the Progressive Care Unit is vacant, workers will begin expanding the NICU into its space, to create one of the largest such neuroscience units in the country, and certainly the largest run entirely by the specialists called neurointensivists.

Rounds begin at 8 a.m., one hour early for a Saturday. The four patients left here in the NPCU, who may be at a slim remove from needing the most careful watch represented by the NICU next door, must be moved to their new locations. The breakdown, already well underway, will run to completion on this, the last day of the hospital year. Beds, monitors, cables, pressure gauges, desks, chairs, carts and charts, reference books and the endless blank forms that become records of patients' lives during their critical days and nights here, all must go. In a fitting closing act, the clock over the nurses' station will be torn from the wall.

The white-coated cluster led by attending physician Mike Williams and followed by Diana Greene-Chandos, the new fellow fresh from Washington University, plus the continuing fellows and residents in neurosurgery and neurology, moves along at what seems a brisk pace past the bed of each patient awaiting a place one floor down.

But the speed is an illusion. The processional stops for twenty minutes or more at each patient's feet. The chart-cart's pace falls in rhythm with the beep of monitors, the hurried passage of nurses, and the doctors' clipped voices that march with the precision of a military band through vital statistics and warning signs. The doctors' and nurses' voices, like a spoken canon interwoven with monitoring sounds and the rattle of wheels, seem to fit the cart's rhythm as they move from room to room.

Hematocrit leads into platelets to be followed by concentrations of sodium and potassium and then PCO_2. By now this is second nature to everyone. Red blood cells, counted by hematocrit, carry oxygen to the brain; they contain platelets, which help blood clot, counted separately in the report. Two numbers, two measures of blood health. Sodium and potassium are key for blood flow, brain-cell communication, and other metabolism, and the carbon dioxide pressure—PCO2—represents the exhaust, vented from the lungs, of the body's metabolic engine.

Patient George R____: "Give him twice the usual IV to build blood volume, and concentrate sodium chloride at 30 ccs. We're doing three things at once here. Volume gives the heart more to work with," says Williams, for R____ is a heart patient with a brain hemorrhage, a common combination that radically increases the challenge. The 69-year-old man must be navigated between rock and whirlpool: some of the drugs that might help his brain bleeding could spell trouble for his heart, and vice versa. But dopamine should work for both problems. "Dopamine"—the chemical that facilitates communication among some brain cells, including those involved in blood-flow control—"will enhance his hemodynamics. And sodium chloride should reduce brain swelling."

Williams, of middle height and medium build, began here as a fellow more than a decade ago. His droll humor surfaces in most conversations with peers and fellows. "This will all be gone soon," he had said a day earlier to Greene-Chandos, the newcomer, wagging a finger. "Don't make any engrams"—scientific jargon for memories. He is precise and compact in every movement of his body language. But with patients, as now, his voice is compassionate, soothing: "We're going to move you down to the stand-in backup unit, okayyy? Someone will be along for you in just a few minutes. Okay, sir? Very good. We'll get you out just as soon as we can."

Williams also cochairs the group that must confront the most difficult questions of critical care, the Hospital Ethics Committee. Its members grapple with everything from end-of-life decisions to protocols for organ donation. Abstract legal and ethical concepts of consciousness and free will, compassion and the saving of lives must be brought to bear on real people and their families, in the most extreme conditions.

On to Wilma J____, who has been quadriplegic for many years but now is suffering from a deadly syndrome with the quaint name Ondine's curse, after the mythical sprite punished with it. Like Ondine, Wilma breathes normally when awake, but her breathing may stop as soon as she falls asleep. She must be kept on a respirator that will breathe for her, just in case.

A young man is next, smiling, alert. He is deemed well enough for the floor, so most of the time is spent writing orders to accompany him. An interesting facet of the Neuro ICU and those whose professional lives are spent here: Once patients are well enough to chat, laugh, be themselves, they're usually quickly gone.

But sometimes appearances are deceiving.

"Good morning! Mr. Brown!" The only time anyone raises a voice in the unit is to get a rise out of someone just over the horizon. The resident now is singing out to an elderly man who was found unconscious on the street last night. "Can you show me your hand? Show me your hand Mr. Brown! Very good! Now, can you tell me where you are, Mr. Brown?"

"What?" Mr. Brown's loud response sounds a bit annoyed. "No! You tell me where I am."

A chuckle. "I want *you* to tell *me* where you are, so I know you know."

"No. I want *you* to tell *me* where I am so *I* know."

So Mr. Brown does not know where he is, but he has just passed a sophisticated test in word play. At that level, his mind is clicking along, whatever else may be missing. The team moves on.

The unit through which they round is carved from a vast corner of the seventh floor of the Meyer Building. The critical care patients' windows face east, with a view across Wolfe Street of the equally tall School of Public Health. But that corner in turn is split into enough spaces that the full size of the unit is hidden. The large nurses' station sits opposite, west of the patient rooms. Then down at the end of the wide corridor, the remainder of the unit sweeps in an L along the south face of Meyer, its family visitor room offering spectacular views of Baltimore's harbor and downtown. Straight down below is the U-shaped drive of the main hospital entrance bordered by the Phipps Clinic, whose Victorian brickwork harks back to the old Johns Hopkins nestled in what then was country on the city's eastern edge. This whole wing will be closed off after today so work crews can tear out its entire infrastructure.

As the team passes Room 762, to visit the final patient next door, the phone begins to ring. And ring. An empty white room, its bed starchy white, its occupant gone—home or to the floor, let's hope. But the room would not likely have remained empty to suggest the question in this busy unit, until today. It's the harbinger of Sunday, tomorrow, when this area will be deserted. Tomorrow, too, Dr. Diana Greene-Chandos will have to shoulder the first-call duty as a new fellow, a burden she and colleague Chere Chase have accepted, as they must. No one would greet it gladly. For their first month, they will once again be treated as residents—the hospital grunts, keeping watch and meeting emergencies through lonesome nights and numbingly busy days. Hopkins requires this of those neurointensive fellows whose residencies were at other hospitals.

But working in extremis is nothing new to Greene-Chandos. That's what she trained for. Tall and willowy with bright red hair, blue eyes, a wide, engaging smile, she would hit the ground running no matter what the circumstances. She had met her husband, Brendan Chandos, when he was chief neurology resident and she was a new resident at the University of Washington in Seattle. They married and she completed her residency, first pregnant, then as a new mother—at Washington University in St. Louis, where Brendan had been hired as an attending physician. She had planned to train there as a neurointensivist with Michael Diringer. Then

Brendan got a job as head of neurology at Baltimore County's St. Agnes Hospital. So she opted for this fellowship. She would be the first fellow to face the grueling two years' training while a mother, her mind already crowded with concerns about day care for 15-month-old Connor as she was beginning her own academic year.

Still, it was a bit disconcerting when a senior colleague had said to her, "Have a nice dinner. Say goodbye to your husband and kids." She had risen at 4:30 a.m. to get here by 6, hitting every red light between I-95 and the hospital. But luckily, as they wheeled a patient along the endless trek to the subterranean MRI suite, a nurse she'd told of her commute offered her a speedy shortcut here from her home in suburban Columbia.

JUNE 30 MARKS MIDYEAR in most of the Western world, but in every teaching hospital in the United States the new year begins tomorrow, July 1, with all the frenzied commotion, confusion, apprehension and insomnia of New Year's Day combined with the first day of school crackling in the air, for it is both. For the Romans, Janus was the god of the new year, his two faces looking forward and back. So he is a good household god for these hospital units devoted to the critical care of the brain, where the litany each morning and evening begins with history and ends with prescription.

Today, the guard changes. Williams rounds out the old year as attending physician; in the morning, Anish Bhardwaj, the NICU's associate director, will open the new. The junior fellow becomes senior; and the senior fellows become assistant professors and colleagues of those 1,810 Hopkins faculty members. Residents will put another annual notch in the passage to their specialties.

Until recently, most neurointensivists have been men. In the new year, for the first time, both of the fellows at Johns Hopkins are women. Mirski and Bhardwaj had brought Diana Greene-Chandos and Chere Chase through the unit yesterday during rounds to introduce them to the medical and nursing staffs. This was the period of manic bustling, mixing sublime and ridiculous, that marks all institutional beginnings. How appropriate then that, after their introductory rounds, Greene-Chandos and Chase had to hurry outside on a pallid, humid morning to join the rest of the team to be photographed in front of Johns Hopkins's most famous landmark, The Dome, for the annual picture "in uniform." And that had required, yet a day earlier, that they hurry out of orientation on essentials like the first-line antibiotics prescribed at this hospital, to be fitted for that uniform: knee-length white coats embroidered in red with their names above Department of Anesthesia and Critical Care Medicine, their home unit.

In a few weeks, that picture will join only one other outside the NICU's administrative office, marking Marek Mirski's short tenure as chief. These pictures represent the building blocks of every unit in American medical academia: the annual white-coated assemblages of trainees and their mentors. Time marks the progress of the trainees, and as they in turn march upward through the ranks, their home departments and their chiefs are judged. So the photos proliferate year by year outside the door of every mentor. The multiple rows of lined-up physicians, whose artless repetitiveness would make a photo editor weep, are vital emblems. What they lack in art, they more than make up for in a message as direct as bars stacked on a graph. The rows of lined up physicians are the academic institute's most important product, their number and achievements the measure of their training.

THE WHITE-COATED TROOP is gone now, so the furniture movers' activities become more overt but are all the more carefully patrolled. Every front-line unit needs a no-nonsense sergeant major. The NICU's is Ski Lower. In her mid-fifties, she is the only nurse manager the Johns Hopkins Neurosciences Critical Care Unit has ever had in its nearly 20 years. For her, "neurointensive" is a way of *nursing* patients, which it largely is by the admissions criteria. This morning she marches along the nearly deserted corridor in pink slacks and a white T-shirt emblazoned with the logo of the Brain Attack Stroke Team. The workers from the office-relocators firm move in the desultory fashion of temps, loading boxes and cellophane packages onto any cart that can be turned into a moving dolly.

"Where you going with that?" Even before she sings out, you know Ski is not one of the regular nurses, not even one of the special breed of neuro nurses she helped create. Her stride is too purposeful, her gaze too all-encompassing and assessing, and there is a clear tone of command in her question. The years have softened her face and the figure that gave her the teenage nickname "Ski," for "Skinny," but she looks in fighting trim. Smiling, she is maternal; frowning, a displeased judge.

"The crash cart should be the last thing that goes," she says, referring to the cart that carries the arsenal of weapons against patients' "coding," including ventilator, defibrillator, and resuscitator. The patients remaining in the unit after rounds are neither the sickest nor the most well, but until the last one is gone, the crash cart must remain. It is not just another moving dolly.

Lower has played a major role in redesigning the new unit, because it is the nurses who are constantly with patients and who are most aware of needs for space, storage, and access to patients and critical information. Now she rounds the bright, deserted wing with an eye on what will be.

"A neuro ICU room has to have, first, good access to the head of the bed. Space for support equipment that will allow access to the patient, for anyone who needs it," she says. "The average nurse is a five-foot, four-inch woman, so that's the relevant height for things. And minimal storage space." She smiles: "Nurses are pack rats. Put in closets and drawers, and they'll be filled with stuff that doesn't need to be there."

Continuing down the hall, imagining the large new rooms: there must be space for a nurse, a physician and—for the frequent emergency of a blocked airway—an anesthesiologist, the master of airway control. But in a teaching hospital, she says with a sigh, "need and want run together. Everyone wants to get into the room, especially the newest resident."

She meets with the architects every week or so, but "I don't trust architects." They don't understand neuro space. "They always tell you what everyone *else* does. But our needs are special. They wanted to put computers in the rooms. First, that takes up space. Second, *clatter clatter clatter* at the keyboard. Our patients need quiet whenever they can get it. And darkness. It has to be possible to completely darken the room." Instead, a computer will be found at each nurse's work station in the corridor, one squeezed between each pair of rooms. One nurse watches over two patients here, compared with four out on the floor.

And what will be in a patient's line of sight? "Artwork, changeable. We'll put up posters overhead and on the walls."

Lower shakes her head over some requirements of the Americans with Disabilities Act, or ADA, whose rules imply that NICU staff themselves might be disabled. "A nurse has to be able to turn on a dime and, in the middle of the night, push a hospital bed alone" all the way to the CT scanner, which is literally blocks from here, underground.

She and a nurse-friend who is disabled regularly shake their heads as they regale one another with some new folly of the inflexible rules. Lower toured another hospital's new emergency room that featured a wheelchair-accessible physicians' toilet, taking up huge amounts of tight space, equipped with braille signage. "Can you imagine a blind trauma surgeon in a wheelchair?" she asks.

The heavy, high-tech monitoring equipment in each room will be suspended from columns dropping from the ceiling, an expensive replacement for the floor posts now in the rooms, but one she believes is worth the cost.

"Those posts have been there for 20 years. They're hard to clean around, and after all that time they get scungey." And the new models will allow for transfer of IV and monitoring equipment from ceiling mounts to rolling-bed mounts, so they can be quickly moved with the patient to the operating room or radiology suite.

More than the physical qualities of this unit, though, Ski has helped create the NICU nurse. She established specialty courses that help neuro nurses advance in expertise, and she now teaches the teachers, lecturing regularly throughout the country. She instituted systems of training and promotion that give nurses tangible rewards for their development. Like tenured faculty, NICU nurses run their own committees governing peer review and education and management issues such as scheduling. She is a member of the Maryland Commission on the Crisis in Nursing, and her views of that pending disaster are tightly woven into her views on training. "Hospital beds close because they don't have nurses to staff them, almost for no other reason," she says. "Nurses leave nursing because they get demoralized, and to prevent that you have to show this generation that an investment in their jobs is an investment in themselves, as professionals." And like all good sergeants major, Lower is intensely proud of her team. "There's no nursing crisis here," she says. "Our nurses don't leave."

Finally, this afternoon, she helps move the bed carrying the last patient from here to Halsted 6. "You know, it's moving day," she tells Wilma
J____, adding of the new digs, "It's not going to be as nice as this. You're
going from the Ritz to a motel."

In the otherwise empty family waiting room hangs a festive crepe-pa-
per bell, a relic of winter holidays now ready for the hospital's New Year.
Tall windows streaming sunlight look out over the old Phipps Psychiatric
Clinic bordering the current main entrance, and farther out toward the
glistening harbor a few miles southeast. By midafternoon only a hand-
drawn sign will be left, alerting everyone that as of 2 p.m. today, NPCU WILL
BE OUT OF BUSINESS here on Meyer 7, directing those who might wander
by to the new home on Halsted 6. THANKS FOR THE MEMORIES. And that's
auld lang syne.

CHAPTER 2

Going Under

July 3, 6:15 a.m.

AREK MIRSKI scans his e-mail, then exits his eighth-floor office past the sign reading DEPARTMENT OF ANESTHESIA AND CRITICAL CARE MEDICINE—the aegis under which his Neurosciences Critical Care Unit now operates. It's a mouthful of a title, a union suggesting intricate relationships, like those arising from the intermarriage of powerful families, breeding both synergy and tension. As director of the Division of Neurological Critical Care as well as the chief of Neuroanesthesia, Mirski has citizenship in both Neurology and Anesthesia, which to some would create conflicting demands but to him is purely a strength.

From the beginning, both Neurology and Anesthesia had administrative roles in the NICU, and that fit the training mission. Cecil Borel, anesthesiologist, had impressed the lessons of critical care from their origin in the operating room, and Hanley had led through the subtle intricacies of the neuro exam and the daunting complexities of diagnosis, as well as the demands of academic research. Then, before Mirski took over, Anesthesia took over all financial administration of Neuro Critical Care. For that, Mirski was grateful. On the purely pragmatic side, in every American medical center, Anesthesia is rich in cash flow and Neurology is poor; but more important, Anesthesia departments tend to be cost effective and businesslike, Neurology so intensely grant-oriented that billing and other critical financial matters often fall by the wayside. Finally, the harmony implied in the division's joint ownership was at least as important to Mirski.

The neurology- and anesthesia-based neurointensivists and the neurosurgeons here work hand in glove. That was the goal from the beginning. By contrast "murderous, malignant competition between neurosurgery, neurology, anesthesia and medicine" hobbles many hospital units, he says. In such overheated environments, decisions are driven underground, so key players learn of them when it's too late to alter course. Secrecy and suspicion lead to more of the same. No more do military-style abrasiveness, domination, and authoritarianism work, to Mirski. For him, the hallmarks of well-run medical units are openness and mutual respect.

Administration will be on Mirski's back burner this week because he is booked solid in the operating room. But his antipathy toward "old school" training will emerge in his teaching style, and, because it's early in the new hospital year, mentoring duties will weave their way into nearly every action Mirski takes today, drawing out the day by incremental insertions so it will stretch beyond twelve hours. He hustles from Meyer 8 down one floor, passes his Neuro ICU, heads north past the Medical and the Surgical ICUs through Osler to Halsted—each building memorializing a founder of its realm.

Mirski is still recovering from hip surgery to correct a joint injured and subsequently misformed in a teenage bicycling injury—an injury that never stopped him from playing football, basketball, or tennis, or from running track at MIT. Even the surgery did not slow his fast walking pace. He is six feet tall and, at 43, athletically slim, with dark brown hair and mustache.

He had taken over the unit just two years ago, ending a period of tension and frustration between Dan Hanley and those who ran the two units in which the NICU was embedded—and between Hanley and the nursing staff, which was at least as serious in terms of keeping things on keel. Mirski had made two major proposals for this year's budget, keeping his fingers crossed that one would be approved and the other looked on with encouragement. Both had been fully funded, without debate.

First, of course, was the major expansion of the Neuro ICU that would create the largest closed unit of its kind in the United States. *Closed,* again, is the key word, because it meant that whatever was built Mirski and his team had to run. Second, his plan was approved for the Hopkins neurointensivists to take over the troubled NICU at Bayview Medical Center, and they had done so on July 1. Hopkins had owned and operated Bayview for most of a decade but had never revised management of its NICU. Suffice to say, for now, that the situation had grown so serious that the nurses had threatened to quit. That would have been the end of the Bayview NICU. Now Romer Geocadin, who completed his training just as Mirski took over as chief, became attending neurointensivist at Bayview, dividing his time between the two hospitals.

The new administrative plan meant another eight beds for the team to manage, and these a few miles away. Managing all of this, allocating attending intensivists, fellows, the rotating residents of neurology and neurosurgery would be a major test of administrative skill. Luckily, Mirski had Ski Lower to coordinate the nursing side of the operation, the most critical for the day-to-day management of patient care. But that his two proposals were approved so readily, as anyone familiar with administration knows, was not merely approbation for Mirski's ideas but a vote of confidence in him, and one that he would have to justify over the coming year.

AT HALSTED 7, HE TURNS RIGHT to enter the vast complex of operating suites where most Johns Hopkins surgeries are performed. There he checks the schedule board for his cases and those of the new residents and fellows he supervises, then dons his neuroanesthesiologist's hat, literally, along with mask and gloves. His cases will run throughout the day. He will break from them as he can, hurrying to meetings and a teaching session in the NICU. Even in a busy teaching hospital, there are few whose schedules are as crowded or whose demands are as diverse as Mirski's.

As July opens this new hospital year, graduate M.D.'s begin their specialty training—residency—in everything from pediatrics to emergency medicine to one of the specialties of the neurosciences, such as brain surgery, neurology or anesthesia. Hopkins's is the largest anesthesia department in the country, new residents were told a few days ago, and the department is in charge of 50 operating rooms here and in other buildings in the medical center cluster. The ORs often run around the clock to meet demand.

The neuroanesthesia procedures posted for Mirski on the daily schedule board run the gamut. There is a brain tumor to be removed. There is a shunt that has become clogged and must be replaced, the shunt draining the cavern-like ventricles in the center of the brain, where cerebrospinal fluid is made. And there will be two operations on the spine, whose cord in neuroscience terms is simply the filamentous extension of brain that innervates every part of the body, inside and out, the wiring of feeling and acting human. Today's cases also represent a spectrum of what is possible and what can go wrong in the brain.

Consider Tammy Brasher, a raven-haired, smiling 31-year-old who gave up her life as a Navy sailor shipping to the Mediterranean and Indian Ocean, to the Gulf during the 1991 war, to have two children she now raises as a single mother—at least until she and fiancé Joe Rose marry this fall. She is so upbeat and alert she could be part of the OR crew, leaning up on her elbows on the gurney as it is wheeled in. She is toughing out her second craniotomy—skull-opening brain surgery—for a particularly dangerous type of brain tumor called an astrocytoma. Neurosurgeon Alessandro Olivi will assess what appears to be regrowth of the tumor. Then, within the cavity left by her first operation, he will insert a "Gliadel wafer," a disk most closely resembling a communion wafer but impregnated with the anticancer drug carmustine. Hopefully, this directly applied chemotherapy source will knock out any cancerous cells remaining.

Brasher's tumor had been discovered by as serendipitous a twist of fate as anyone could imagine. She and Joe, ardent Baltimore Ravens fans, were leaving a game against the Steelers last fall when a melee broke out. Tammy was knocked down and either knocked out or coincidentally passed out. Either way, it was a lucky blow. A CT scan disclosed the tumor before she'd had any symptoms, and she had been "adopted" by the team as she went through her treatment.

"Hi, I'm Dr. Mirski." Said in the level, unwavering, somewhat nasal voice that never changes pitch, under any circumstances. "I'll be managing your anesthesia here this morning. I'll be with you every step of the way, and I'll see you later in the recovery room."

"You bet," she says. Two residents accompany Mirski this morning, and she eyes them a bit suspiciously. "Are they students?"

"There are no students here," he says. "I'm the Neuroanesthesia division leader, and my job is taking them to my level—which won't be hard, given how good they are."

"Good," she says brightly. "I'm going to get well quickly. I have two little ones at home."

Mirski is right about the residents, of course, in the fundamental sense of "student." But Brasher's perception is not entirely off the mark. All residents are full-fledged physicians who have undergone a further year of post-graduate internship. Additionally, both residents this morning had completed several years' residency training in other specialties before switching to anesthesia. But the first week of the hospital year is a grueling one for attendings like Mirski, residents, and fellows alike because even well-learned lessons must be repeated, and repeated again. In a sense, as at no other time of the year, everyone is a student, a mentor, or alternately both. It is a time, according to medical legend, when far more mistakes are made than at any other time of the year, and more serious mistakes, to boot. That belief was challenged recently by a study offering evidence that the truth is almost the reverse—that the riskiest week of the year statistically is the last in June, perhaps because concentration shifts more toward changes to come rather than cases at hand. Nevertheless, one thing is clear. So intent is everyone on not becoming an anecdote in the grim legend that July is a wonderful time for an observer to lurk, to hear everything explained to the fullest, and to hear the reasons behind policies that newcomers want to know, however well-trained they may have been elsewhere.

Although Tammy Brasher's case may be a hopeful one, there are no growths in the brain that are truly benign, as they can be elsewhere in the body. Brain tumors do not have to grow large or spread beyond their territory to kill, unlike most deadly cancers. The brain is so susceptible to pressure and its smallest territories are so eloquent that some tumors can be fatal even when the immune system encapsulates them, in defense against their spread. Like most brain tumors, Brasher's comes from improper growth of one of the support cells for neurons, the neurons being the firing, communicating units we think of as "brain cells." The support cells—such as the astrocytes of Brasher's tumor—actually compose most of the brain's mass. The good news for Tammy is that her tumor was on the right side, in her frontal lobe, and was neither large nor growing fast. Most people's language abilities derive from the left hemisphere, thus it is the more dangerous side for surgery. And although motor skills are located on both sides—the left controlling the right side of the body and vice versa—Tammy's were untouched by her earlier surgery so should not be affected now.

Within minutes, explaining each step as he goes, Mirski has injected Brasher's intravenous wrist catheter with a sedative that renders her drowsy, listless. Then another shot puts her to sleep, and at that point he holds the mask of inhalational gas over her face. When he judges her at the right depth of anesthesia, he removes the mask and stands behind her head with the curved metal intubation cylinder, or laryngoscope. While holding her neck up with one hand, he smoothly slips the tube into her mouth, around the curve of her throat, and down. It is one of the smoothest, simplest actions to watch in emergency medicine, and one of the more difficult to master. Mirski's narrative as he performs it is not on how-to, which the residents know, but on the importance of balancing and smoothly shifting their weight to conserve their energy for a long day.

The inhalational gases now will be fed through this tube. In critical care terms, the tube has given him control of her airway, next to heartbeat the most critical life process that must be sustained at all times. She is breathing on her own, though at a far lower rate than when conscious. But if something went wrong, Mirski and his team could begin artificially breathing for her within seconds, with a ventilator.

The next 20 minutes are consumed with insertions of catheters by the anesthesiologists and nurses. There is an A line into the radial artery in the wrist, measuring blood pressure there. A central line, much tougher to place, goes into the superior vena cava, the large vein just above the heart, where it will measure pressure inside the right atrium as blood returns to the heart. And finally, the balloon-like Swann-Ganz catheter is carefully fed through the heart and into the giant pulmonary artery pumping the oxygen-depleted blood from the heart into the lungs for recharging.

Swirling around the inert form, the gowned, masked figures bring all the technology of modern medicine to as tight a focus on the patient here as a deity might get in a religious ritual. The OR is the birthplace of neurological intensive care, the nearby Neuro ICU representing an extension of the obsessive scrutiny of brain function pioneered here.

As surgery rapidly developed in the early twentieth century with the advent of safer anesthetics, sterile operating rooms, and better surgical techniques, it became apparent that no one among the many physicians typically engaged in the procedure was in charge of the patient. The anesthesiologist, in Dan Hanley's words, became the patient's advocate in the operating room, the first and final case manager, in theory over even the surgeon in control of the patient. Mirski and crew are like ships' pilots, who take operational command from captains when vessels enter harbor channels.

In turn, many of the life-saving monitoring and rescuing techniques of the operating room were developed in cardiovascular surgery, whose frontiers are considered to be 20 years ahead of neuro's, and were extended to the intensive care of heart patients. That lag time speaks partly to the unfathomable complexities of the brain, the unpredictable ways its vessels and structures can respond counter to all data, and the devastating outcomes when things go wrong. The heart is a beautiful machine, a wondrous muscle that can beat without rest for a century and more. But there is no analogy for what the brain is like. A brain is like nothing else except other brains, and nowhere near identical to any of them.

As accomplished as these anesthesia residents are, Mirski automatically talks through many of his procedures, citing research articles, comparing drug efficacies, rattling off long branches of "if, then, otherwise" scenarios. While neurosurgeon Olivi focuses every bit of his attention on the tiny vessels that loom at him through the intraoperative microscope, Mirski or his assistant constantly monitors the human beneath layers of sheeting, bandage, and adhesive. If something goes wrong inside that must be treated "emergently," the anesthesiologist holds nearly all the tools and will take charge.

Sometimes, when surgery is planned close to a critical cranial nerve or control area, Mirski will monitor evoked potentials. It's a simple but fascinating procedure in which an electrical signal is sent to check the brain's circuitry; the healthy brain signals back. Is the surgeon operating near the motor region that controls moving the right index finger? Then an electrical pulse delivered at the proper spot on the left motor strip should make the right index finger move. Or is this operation near the brain region that senses what the right index finger feels? Then a stimulus to the right finger must show a pulse of monitor activity from the left sensory region. No response means danger.

Major risks of surgery to be watched for: sudden changes in blood pressure that will call for counter-balancing drugs; hemorrhage that might or might not require anticoagulants, massive transfusion of new blood, or both; changes in heartbeat.

Mirski tells the new residents that the watchwords of their profession are *steadiness* and *organization*. "When neurosurgeons see that my name is on the case," he says, "I want them to breathe easier—with complete confidence that they can focus entirely on their job, because I will be in control—and know that if things were to get out of control, I would regain control or help them regain control."

Control, repeated as regularly as a mantra, is the common goal in both the operating room and the intensive care unit. Surprise is the enemy, for it implies lost control and an immediate threat to the patient. So the prayer, sometimes uttered, otherwise tacit, is for order, quiet, and predicted response, especially for those in their first weeks here on call. Of course, at some point, at some time, *control will be lost.* That's the nature of the activity in the OR and illnesses in the ICU. When it is lost, it must be regained at minimal cost to the patient, but regained at all costs, and that's what everyone is training for.

And as mentor, of course, he must also prepare residents for the harrowing specialty-certification boards, where they will be bombarded with horrific scenarios of disaster in the OR, to which they will have to respond immediately and correctly.

Mirski advises: "On your boards, don't try to sit and think what you'd do in the described situation. Picture yourself standing right where you are. The patient crashes. You know what to do, you've done it many times: this and this and this to gain control of the patient. You don't need to think, you need to see yourself here, doing it. Tell them as though you are *doing* these things as you answer."

Once the wafer is placed in Brasher's brain, the chief neuroanesthesia resident replaces Mirski, who slips through a narrow connecting door to scrub out, immediately scrub in, and enter the adjoining operating room. Once again, this time with a back-surgery patient: "Good morning! Good morning! I'm Dr. Mirski. . . . "

Now the potential dangers change completely. Back surgery is typically less life threatening than operations involving invasion of the skull. But spinal surgery often entails massive blood loss, even when all goes well, because the marrow of vertebral bones is so rich with the blood it produces. Today, for example, Mirski anticipates the patient "losing" four to six liters of blood of the eight liters circulating in his body. Transfusing replacement blood, making sure enough is on hand, is his job. "You don't want to have to interrupt a surgery while you chase down more blood," he says. "That would mean prolonging anesthesia, which is risky in itself."

But if the neuroanesthesiologist's patient contact is immediate and focused, ordinarily it is brief. "We tend to be nomads," one had said. "We don't see patients in offices, so most of us don't even have offices except as billing addresses. We can move among hospitals without much attachment."

For those who are also neurointensivists, however, everything changes. Mirski is one of relatively few physicians who not only might be the last to soothe patients as they go under and first to greet them in recovery, but he might appear yet again in the intensive care unit, where many post-surgical patients spend at least a first night. "I'm Dr. Mirski, and I'm in charge of the Neuro ICU this week." For in addition to spending two days of most weeks in the operating room, Mirski takes his turn one full week out of every three as attending neurointensivist in charge of the NICU. That means he is on call nights and weekends. A year ago it was tougher. Because of heavy faculty shortages resulting from cutbacks and freezes a few years earlier, Mirski had operating room duty a full week at a time. As head of the division, of course, he has overall administrative charge all the time.

CHAD ARENT, THE PATIENT who rounds out today's cases, carries his story in the lines of his scalp. The chief resident assisting neurosurgeon Daniele Rigamonti shaves the young man's dark hair for a procedure that is as routine as neurosurgery gets, a "shunt revision." But instead of seeing the usual skin-toned, smooth scalp laid bare by the razor, they behold scores and ridges, old suture tracks and incision marks, as well as the thin ridgeline of the shunt tube that is their goal.

One April day four years ago, Chad Arent, 20, celebrated being named kicker for Alabama's Crimson Tide by visiting a girl in another state, a long, hard drive away. Returning home just before dawn, he may have fallen asleep or may have suffered a tire blowout. His truck crashed end over end, so hard that Chad was ejected out of his seatbelt through the back window. The trauma surgeon who first saw him told the Arents he had never seen an accident victim survive with his skull broken in so many places. But maybe that had saved him. "Brain swelling might have killed him if the broken skull hadn't provided room" for the brain to expand, his mother recalls being told.

The shunt is part of the years-long response to that swelling. It drains the brain's vast central ventricles, which in turn drain into the spinal canal. In the ventricles—"vents" in hospital jargon—cerebrospinal fluid is made. The CSF both cushions the surrounding brain and carries off dead brain cells and other waste. If too much fluid is made, it can crush the delicate brain from within. On the other hand, if the brain swells for other reasons, draining fluid to shrink the ventricles can create life-saving room. Shunting the CSF from ventricles into the peritoneum or the lower spinal canal offers a means of rescue. Now Chad's shunt had become infected, a not uncommon occurrence.

A resident who has spoken with the family tells how Michael and Sharon Arent have taken Chad to many rehabilitation centers, now care for him at home. They have, in fact, moved into the basement of their Virginia home and have created a one-patient rehab center.

Mirski listens attentively and says, "Those are the real heroes of the world, right there. I'm not saying it doesn't take courage to stand up and face fire in combat, but to get up in the morning and have the courage to face whatever is coming in this kind of situation is my idea of real heroism. There are so many like that we see here."

Here on the operating table, Chad marks the starting point of a long foray into brain "climate" from the perspective of the pressures it exerts and those to which it must respond. Seeing how the brain works, even at a lay level, requires many journeys from entirely different starting points, along such different pathways that the word *brain* seems their only link.

Dealing with intra-cranial pressure—ICP—would be the first topic Mirski would discuss with the new neurointensivist fellows, whether prompted by Chad or simply part of an annual routine. The junior fellows, Chere Chase and Diana Greene-Chandos, at this moment were awaiting him in the NICU break room for a teaching session.

Mirski leaves his chief anesthesia resident in charge and hurries to the unit, not 50 yards from the operating suites. Out in the hall he works his way through a turmoil of green scrubs outside the two dozen ORs in this main cluster, where members of teams scrub in and out, check the schedule board and converse. That schedule, so vital to the surgeons waiting with their cases, is developed and controlled by the Anesthesia Department, making the department a common center of friction over pecking order and priority.

He heads back to his office, as always on the double, to grab research-journal reprints he will hand the new fellows—for a fellowship this is, in every sense. Chase and Greene-Chandos have not been *hired* to supple-ment the faculty members in Neurointensive Care. They have been *ad-mitted* to begin the long path to become faculty themselves, and hiding behind the frenzy of overnight call and rounds and medical emergency is a powerfully heavy research demand that each will have to confront. For both, research would provide the biggest challenge in the year ahead. Like the dark matter thought to compose so much of the universe, the re-search requirements of a hospital like Johns Hopkins are hidden from view by the glare of the immediate. The rounds. The meetings. The crises. But hidden or not, the demands of research are decisive.

Consider Mirski's curriculum vitae—a model resume for Johns Hopkins, or he wouldn't have this job. After graduating from MIT, he spent the usual six years earning his combined M.D./Ph.D. degrees at St. Louis's Washington University, finally completing a prolonged thesis with an exciting discovery about seizures that promises to change treatment for some forms of epilepsy. He studied how seizures emanate from the core of the brain in guinea pigs to simultaneously devastate multiple sites in the neuronal cortex, at the "thinking" brain surface. He published exten-sively on his model of seizure genesis, and that became the basis for a clinical trial now under way at several major medical centers. He spent a further six years in internship, residency in two specialties—neurology and anesthesia—and then went through his own neurointensive fellow-ship for two years. During residency, he became a father and traded in his two-seater car for the stick shift Subaru station wagon he still drives. Fourteen years of post-graduate training after MIT, he became a junior faculty member at Johns Hopkins in 1993. His salary was $30,000 a year.

For all this, and his four years founding and leading the Neuro ICU in Hawaii, he returned to head this unit as an associate professor. Will he ever make full professor? That will depend to a large degree on decisions he will make in the coming year—decisions on how to shoehorn topflight research into his administrative and clinical agenda. Hopkins promotion committees weigh research at 80 percent of a candidate's effort and count the exhausting clinical duties, with their daily rounds and night calls, at only 20 percent.

However, much as the Mirski C.V. reflects Johns Hopkins, the Mirski personality may be a reaction to its aura. In a world of power lunches, he most often sips microwave noodle soup, feet up in his office—where he now rumages for those reprints—chatting with fellows or colleagues as they too brown-bag. Amid the formality of academic medicine, he often hustles down the halls with a Tootsie Pop stuck in his cheek. Point to it and he will offer you one, or M&Ms from one of several dispensers in his office. Or, his favorite, Peppermint Patties kept chilled in the refrigerator.

Mirski's office reflects the man. His two daughters smile from desk photos. Kara just turned 12 in March, Erin 10 in April. His wife, Lenore Tomoye Nii, M.D., gave up her pediatrics practice to spend more time with their daughters. Gifts from the girls—the M&M dispenser, handwritten poems—dot the large inner office enclosed behind the reception area at the division's entrance. He sits between two parallel desks, the mahogany executive-standard facing south toward the front office, where he can greet visitors, a plain table facing the north wall, holding his computer and reference books and covering the filing cabinet. Between the desks and the entrance is a couch—there you might sit opposite him to talk. More important, the couch will open into his bed on the many nights he spends on call in the OR. Closest to the front office is a small conference table where there might be conferences, but more often of residents and fellows or faculty and their visitors than of Mirski the division head. He is in and out, mostly out. No teacher could be more peripatetic yet so close to "home base." From the OR to the Neuro ICU to meetings elsewhere in the Hopkins complex and back again, passing through his office, touching base and gone.

Once an avid backpacker and outdoorsman, Mirski decided when he returned from Hawaii that the intense pressures of the new duties would not accommodate work, family, and backpacking. So the backpacking went. Work and family is it. He has just returned from two weeks vacationing with Lenore and the girls. They flew to San Francisco, then drove north to spend time with her parents and family, who have lived in the same area of California for four generations. He will think about his earlier career decisions often during the coming year as he considers his future development. Scientist, clinician, administrator. All of the above, or narrow the focus? The only thing he knows for sure, at any given moment, is that he is at center a clinician—a doctor. Sometimes he thinks it would be neat just to be a small-town doctor, a member of local committees, greeted on the street.

Reprints in hand, he's off again.

To many who do not know him well, Mirski seems easygoing, dispassionate. But that manner is belied by the intensity of his schedule, his discussion of the issues the neurointensivists face, the drive that lies behind his daily and career choices. He began in neurology, but then came the now-familiar moment of awakening: "I was frustrated I couldn't do enough. I wanted to get in the game, to intervene aggressively." He decided that residencies in both neurology and anesthesia would give him both the skills to care for the toughest cases and the diagnostic abilities to read the critical events within the brain.

And driving him, too, is the legacy of his parents. He had only recently reflected, he said to Lenore, that "a lot of what I do is a desire to pay back their expectations." Both Jerzy and Janina Mirski were heroes of the World War II Polish Resistance as teenagers, surviving the harrowing collapse of

Warsaw at war's end. Both went on to important professional careers, Jerzy getting a Ph.D. in economics and Janina a master's in civil engineering after they immigrated to Washington, D.C. There, Marek and his younger sister, Eva, were born and grew up. Janina became a prominent figure in designing hospitals to withstand earthquakes. Both Jerzy and Janina had died within the past couple of years, and he still felt that loss sharply.

Later, in another context, their story would strike me as a parable of predictability, so critical to science, and of the limits of vision as opposed to seeing. Those limits lie somewhere in the brain.

MIRSKI AND CODIRECTOR ANISH BHARDWAJ and fellows Chere Chase and Diana Greene-Chandos sit squeezed around a small table in the break room at the center of the Neuro ICU, gazing at the whiteboard, truly gathered around the brain. "It's encased in a skull, bone that is for all intents and purposes absolutely rigid," Mirski begins. "So there is no room for any of the skull contents to expand." Whatever space one element tries to expand into is taken at the expense of another, he says. Whatever pressure is exerted by one element, must be surrendered by another. "What are those contents?"

Answers from the fellows. First, there is brain itself, the most delicate and least able to suffer contraction without damage. Then, of course, the blood coursing through all the complex territories, its vessels delineated all the way from the huge major arteries, looking like cables under the intraoperative microscope, down to the microscopic capillaries. The capillaries branch so fine that the terminals of single support cells like the astrocytes can wrap around them, their feet forming tight junctures with the lining of the vessels. The tightly bound double layer—brain astrocyte to membrane of the tiniest blood vessel—forms a fascinating wall called the blood-brain barrier that runs throughout the vast territory of the brain. Though discovered more than a century ago, until recent years the blood-brain barrier was mysterious in both its functions and its dysfunctions. And finally, in the triumvirate competing for space within the brain, there is the cerebrospinal fluid bubbling out of a layer of the ventricles called the choroid plexus.

Brain pressure plus blood pressure plus CSF pressure. If volume of one goes up, thus increasing pressure, volume and pressure of the others must go down. Here is the first and among the most complex of the juggling acts in which neurointensivists must engage around the clock. If the brain swells because water has built up within its tissues, that will tend to drive down cerebral blood pressure. If you simply administer drugs to drive the pressure up to keep vital blood-oxygen pumped into brain cells, you may crush the brain tissue in the process. But if an area of the brain becomes oxygen-starved for long enough, it dies. Such death is called infarction—a stroke, of the ischemic variety since no blood vessel has broken. If you go overboard forcing blood pressure higher to meet brain demand, a blood vessel may rupture. The cells downstream from it, like tender shoots in an irrigation channel, will lose oxygen. Infarction type two: stroke of the hemorrhagic variety.

—Unless you drain some CSF. Or you find a way to get the water out of the brain. Bhardwaj is a leading investigator into just this nest of problems, seeking to master the ways fluid can be moved around and pressures adjusted in this most eloquent territory. When someone has a stroke, what causes the damage? What seems like a simple question with an easy answer—lost oxygen from interrupted blood supply—is in fact both complex and absorbing.

Mannitol is a chemical—a sugar—that removes water from the brain, so it is a major part of the arsenal against brain swelling. But plain salt water, in Bhardwaj's words, "literally sucks water out of the brain," just as salt poured on a snail will suck the water from its tissues, leaving it shriveled. In everyday English, you pump salt water into the brain; in medical terms, you administer hypertonic saline intravenously. Bhardwaj prefers salt water to mannitol and other medications, for reasons he has been researching and publishing extensively over many years.

Make the rounds any morning or evening and you will hear, body system by body system, machine-gun bursts of numbers—data points on the patient's life chart—and corresponding return bursts of pharmaceuticals to be fired back, to boost this, lower that. In the NICU, one whole category of numbers is parsed for one kind of information: those three pressures in the skull. And one or more orders written in response may be aimed at balancing this triad. Brain pressure. Blood pressure. CSF pressure.

The new fellows, of course, have heard this all before, through three years' residency in neurology following four years medical training and a year's internship, but they brought their knowledge to Baltimore with very different perspectives. When Greene-Chandos trained with Diringer at Washington University, mannitol was the order of the day.

Diringer loves mannitol, fast-acting, long-lived in the blood. "We probably use more mannitol here than anyone," he said recently. Like salt, mannitol sucks water from the brain. Unlike salt, it breaks down the blood-brain barrier. What does that mean? The blood-brain barrier is evolution's answer to the brain's need for exquisitely controlled chemical balances. What the brain requires, it admits in an inactive, safer form, converting these few precursors into the dozens of active molecules it needs, in just the quantities, at just the places and just the moments it needs them. Most chemicals, thus most drugs, cannot get into the brain. Most of the time, that's terrific. But it makes the brain tough to medicate. Sometimes you need to prize apart the tight junctions of the brain's capillaries just a touch, to squeeze in some life-saving drug molecules. Mannitol does that, as well as reducing swelling.

And that's why Bhardwaj doesn't like it. By disrupting the blood-brain barrier, mannitol admits more than just the desired drug, and that "more" can be mischief. Except when absolutely needed, Bhardwaj eschews mannitol in favor of a plain salt solution. Bhardwaj and Diringer: two senior neurointensivists, trained in the same program; two divergent views of one of the most common tools to alleviate swelling in the brain, and each finding ways to make his choice work "best."

Greene-Chandos and Chase, side by side as their NICU training begins, will become good friends this year, a year that will test their mettle in ways that define *unpredictable*. They come to this from far different professional and family backgrounds, and even their expectations for the years following their training diverge. At the moment, Greene-Chandos envisions herself becoming the first woman to complete fellowship training while mothering a small child, perhaps even having another. Chase foresees herself as the first African-American woman to be fellowship-trained as a neurointensivist, anywhere. Greene-Chandos hails from a traditional "nuclear" family in Scottsdale, Arizona. Chase grew up in suburban New Jersey, her single-parent mother a bank executive whose drive, intelligence, and zeal inspired her daughter to excel at every endeavor. Chase remembers being perhaps not chastised but cautioned over every B on her report card. "There *are* three medals in the Olympics," Joyce Chase always acknowledged. "But only one of them is gold."

Initially Greene-Chandos and Chase had seriously contemplated stepping right into the neurointensive fellowships at their residency institutions, where both programs were run by Hanley trainees. That was Diringer at Wash U for Greene-Chandos. For Chase, it was the Cleveland Clinic, as famous for "brain medicine" as Johns Hopkins; she considered staying there with José Suarez, her neurology mentor and a top neurointensivist. Chase's boyfriend lives in Cleveland, and the drive is far shorter from there to Pittsburgh, where her mother and grandmother live, than from Baltimore. Neurointensive care attracted her not least because of its income potential, which generally is quite low for neurologists among the medical specialties but is better for subspecialties in demand. Long term, Chase decided, the Johns Hopkins brand on her curriculum vitae would be far more marketable, especially outside the Midwest. So here she came.

But from this beginning the two fellows' paths would now diverge sharply, right through the year's conclusion. First off, Greene-Chandos had a smooth, quiet opening week of call. Everything stayed under control.

CHAPTER 3

The Will to Die

A SLOW WEEK in the Neuro ICU. Less than a day out of the OR, Tammy Brasher worked her way from intensive care to "the floor," up two flights. On Wednesday morning, twelve hours postop, she sits up in bed, blankets tucked around her and legs crossed, as though gabbing with friends at a sleepover. She is expecting her fiancé Joe Rose at any moment with her children, Krystal, 8 , and Michael, 7.

Most people are groggy and sluggish after the deep anesthesia of neurosurgery, she is told.

"Not me. Don't have time for it. I'll be back to work in three weeks," she says brightly. She has a degree in financial business administration from Penn State she earned while in the Navy and is an administrator at a local architectural firm. "They set up a computer for me to work at home, but I won't be there long."

Her neurosurgeon is optimistic about her chances, she says. "Olivi told me I'm on my way to a full and complete recovery." But her oncologist had not been so positive about the ability of the wafer implant to completely kill her brain cancer. "I was told I had 12 to 18 months to go. I didn't believe it then and I don't believe it now."

Stuck here this Fourth of July, she sees a bright side. "Everybody says the fireworks in the harbor are great to watch from the family waiting room here," she says. "So we'll have the kids come and watch them." It's a warm image: Tammy, Joe, and the kids gathered before the great window looking off toward the bay, and she a fine match for Mirski's definition of a *hero*.

It has been a dry, cool summer so far, especially so by the standards of humid Baltimore. This morning dawned the same, but over the afternoon the sky goes gray, by losing light. Clouds do not move in—they materialize all around, like an enveloping mood. About 5 p.m. rain starts, while the surrounding air is still full of light, as though it had been trapped below; the buildings shine with a patina as they soak. In the evening, lightning streaks and flashes through the dark sky. Fireworks of a natural sort, a grim prognosis for the downtown display that must have been washed out along with Tammy's plans. Not so. The fireworks started after the end of visiting hours, but the nurses lifted the rule, this once; the show was spectacular and they all had a great time.

LATE FRIDAY AFTERNOON, Anish Bhardwaj got a strange call from the emergency room at Maryland General Hospital, across town—that is, the case he was asked to triage had unusual elements. Calls to evaluate the seriousness and best critical-care specialty to handle an emergency were commonplace when neuro status was an issue. A young man named Jay Lokeman had been brought in by police on a call to a downtown retirement home, where he had apparently suffered a seizure in the parking lot. But then he had wrestled the police all the way to the hospital, where tranquilizers finally calmed him down. Regaining consciousness, he had tried to tell the admitting physician he'd simply had a fall, whether because he could remember nothing else or was anxious to be released was impossible to tell. But then his blood work showed Lokeman to be dangerously septic. He was full of infection, and of more than one type.

When Bhardwaj examined him, his skin was mottled and pale, leading him to suspect that the cause might be the frightful necrotizing fasciitis, the misnamed "flesh-eating bacteria" of news reports, which destroys— but does not devour—muscle and underlying tissue. It can kill its victims in days if not controlled. Nevertheless, nothing but the seizure, now past, suggested Lokeman as a candidate for the Neuro ICU, so Bhardwaj suggested that the trauma team admit him into the Medical ICU.

But the seizures returned, subsided, returned again, and then extended into the particularly dangerous stage called *status epilepticus*. So it was the Neuro ICU after all. Once he was there, however, they got him under control and on a major course of antibiotics. He came in too late to be seen on rounds, but Bhardwaj alerted Chase and, in any case, Lokeman seemed calm and well controlled—exhausted, the usual state of a seizure victim— but not in any great danger, other than from the infections. Lokeman's family arrived, he slept, and his first night passed uneventfully. If all went well, Lokeman would be out of the unit in a few days and onto the floor, where he would be kept on intravenous antibiotics for as long as it took to heal his infections.

C H E R E   C H A S E walked through the unit on Saturday, the last day of her first week's call, with the certainty and confidence that marked her every move. In both speech and body language she is precise, concise, direct and focused—at least while in the unit—an attractive, buxom woman who carries herself with cool authority. She can explode with laughter at a good joke once out of the NICU, but with patients she is appropriately cool and collected—though, she always says, the day she doesn't cry when a patient dies, she'll quit practicing medicine. She is very conscious and proud of her heritage, the African-American banker's daughter, potentially the first to complete a fellowship in neurointensive care. She knows that another black woman is a neuro critical care physician at Case Western Reserve in Cleveland, but that woman trained outside this subspecialty. Chase would be the first completed fellow.

For her this first week had an added burden and special reward. Her family—mother and grandmother—had come to spend the week with her. They'd gotten to take in some good movies and just hang together. Pittsburgh, where both lived, was a tiring six-hour drive from Baltimore, compared with only two hours from Cleveland during residency and just a jog down the road from the University of Pittsburgh, where she had done her internship. But at least with them here this first week, she could give them time and still devote herself fully to her duties without having to spend hours on the road as well.

This was the family to whom she owed everything, starting with the work ethic passed from grandmother, still a private-duty nurse at 80, to mother to daughter. Joyce Chase had dropped out of New York University at 19 to get married, then returned to Bloomfield College in New Jersey while Chere was in high school. Joyce graduated magna cum laude and soon become a vice president of her bank, relocating to Pittsburgh when the headquarters moved there. Chere took her string of report card "golds" to Brown University, the Ivy League. She'd owed that achievement to her mother, too. But Chere had a diversity of interests beyond the biology she'd majored in. She went to work for McDonald's as a business trainee at its headquarters, having her mother's strong interest in finance, and considered remaining in business management.

It didn't take long for medicine to draw her back. She refocused an early interest in it by coming to Johns Hopkins for a master's in health science. It was a lucky move, for it made her an in-state resident for tuition purposes two years later, when she enrolled in the University of Maryland medical school, downtown. The drill at Maryland was wonderful because it forced medical students from the very beginning of clinical training to take overnight call, which few other schools did. By the time she became a neurology resident in Cleveland, she knew she could handle the pressure, independence, and exhaustion of call, which was taking many of her contemporaries by surprise.

But in between, the world had turned upside down, in the most unexpected, cruelest way Chere could imagine it. The Christmas of her first med-school year she had given her mother a cassette tape to play in her car while commuting. Joyce had insisted the car, which she'd had for years, had no cassette player, which, of course, it did. And when they went to play the tape together, Joyce could not figure out how to put the cassette into the slot. That was all, memorable only because it was the first sign. Then there were other obvious things Joyce could not remember, coming in quick succession. And then the diagnosis: at only 55 years old, Joyce Chase had Alzheimer's disease.

The banker who would accept nothing less than the gold standard could no longer balance her checkbook. Bill collectors were at her door over many-times forgotten debts; other bills were paid three, four times. Daughter's efforts to take over money management had been strenuously rebuffed. Three weeks ago, after a lifetime of intellectually challenging work, Joyce Chase had retired on disability at age 61. Alzheimer's is often characterized as cruel to families but kind to its victims, who usually are unaware of their deficits. Not this time. Joyce was frustrated and angry, unable to understand why she could no longer do the simple, precise things out of whose threads she had woven her life, their lives. The day Joyce Chase came home from work with a less-than-top evaluation, her speech was slurred and her heart hammered with anxiety. She had had to spend a night in a nearby emergency room, her head splitting with pain.

Now Chere would have to be there. She would support the three of them and pay off the mountain of medical school debt that was the common lot of most graduated physicians. In fact, she would have to begin paying back those loans this year. Held in abeyance through residency, the debts come due during fellowships or any further medical training period. No matter, where there's a will, there's a way, and Chere most certainly had the will.

As everyone knows, in old adventure movies the serene calm of a summer night is a very bad sign. In the stereoptypical scene, someone usually says, "It's quiet out there." Then, blooey, all hell breaks loose. So the resident on first call prays for quiet but is careful not to speak of it, because that would be a provocation and sure to bring bad luck. Chase likes to refer to it as "dancing before the call gods." *Looks like an easy night tonight,* you might say foolishly. Then, blooey. But with mother and grandmother spending their last days before boarding the bus back to Pittsburgh, Chase might have been forgiven for almost tasting the end of her first turn on resident's call, just 12 hours from now at 9 a.m., Sunday. Among the more serious cases there was Wilma J＿＿ and George R＿＿, who had been in the unit for more than a week and were stable. And there was Jay Lokeman, admitted yesterday.

Lokeman might have scared the wits out of many residents with his status epilepticus, but, for Chase, he symbolized the confidence that grew in a physician over the long, trying days and nights of residency training. At the Cleveland Clinic, Hopkins-trained José Suarez had often led her through the complexities of "status," as it is usually shortened to, and cases far worse than this. For now, Lokeman's status seemed under control, not uncommon for a case induced by drug use.

Status epilepticus is an often deadly magnification of a seizure. At a lay level, a seizure is not hard to understand. "To a hammer, everything is a nail," the saying goes. At the level of the single neuron, only one message is received or delivered in the brain: "Fire!" or "Don't fire!" The neuron gets input signals from perhaps a thousand other neurons, some—excitatory—telling it to fire, others—inhibitory—telling it not to fire. If it gets enough positive commands, it fires, and the message it sends to its downstream neuron follows the same rule. It signals "Fire!" if it, the sender, is excitatory, "Don't fire!" if it is inhibitory. No matter how many billions of times multiplied, or across how many chain reactions of cerebral fireworks, the brain's individual cells either fire, or they hold their fire, in response to those incoming signals. It's as binary an action as that at any computer-chip junction. On, off. Fire, don't fire.

Simple seizures are thought to result from a loss of "Don't fire" signals. In a usually small network of cells, inhibition of firing is lost or overcome so that cells fire repeatedly and can recruit other cells to join them. But that lasts for only seconds, a few minutes at most, and then the sufferer recovers, often dazed or semiconscious and exhausted by the surge.

The Latin phrase *status epilepticus* translates literally as "state of epilepsy." As dangerous as seizures can be, they are usually transient. Status epilepticus represents firings in too-quick succession for the brain cells to recover; at worst, the firings of status epilepticus can be endless and fatal.

The western wildfires of this summer of 2001 offered an analogy, on a giant scale, to Lokeman's problem. Conditions from Montana to New Mexico had turned a third of America's forests and rangeland to tinder, upping the odds that small blazes would break out here and there, and that once burning they would grow larger. Add a touch of wind, and you now had good odds that some small fires would join up, or that their wind-driven intensity would consume fuels ordinarily too moist or dense to burn. That was Jay's brain, likely the result of drug abuse.

Perhaps several seizure patterns induced by long use of heroin and cocaine had joined into a "state of fire," blowing out of the small eruptions of brain cells that mark single seizures. Perhaps craving had set off a feedback loop of excitation. Status epilepticus has a huge mortality rate, but it usually can be controlled with antiseizure medications. The medications hit all the fire sites at once like a massive blanket of slurry across the sheet of the cerebral cortex. And if these medications failed, there were more drastic measures Chase had learned to take.

In her three years as a neurology resident she had seen many patients with status epilepticus brought to a safe harbor. She felt comfortable contemplating the treatment course for Lokeman. If his seizures resumed and nothing else worked, the barbiturate pentobarbital would put him in a temporary coma, quieting his brain. Then after a brief time they would lift the barbs and watch. His status should soon be at an end. He would be exhausted by his ordeal, quiet. As long as the pentobarbital could be dosed up without interfering with heart function, he would recover from the status. And Lokeman should be the toughest case she faced tonight.

After rounding on her patients, she headed down the hall, Meyer to Osler to Halsted, to meet with families in the now-crowded waiting room they had to share with the other critical care units, because their own at the west end of the Neuro ICU had closed a week ago.

And while she was there, everything unraveled. Chase got a page from
Holli Takahashi, Lokeman's nurse, urging her to come quickly. Lokeman
had come to, but he was incredibly agitated, thrashing dangerously in an
uncontrolled rage.

Pandemonium greeted her. Lokeman was trying to pull out the tube
in his throat, an agonizing action that might have knocked another patient flat. But in the wild places of his unconscious, in the state wrought
by seizure, drugs and infection, everyone was trying to kill him. Chase
knew that. From his most primitive brain stem upward, Lokeman was a
human animal in a fight for his life, in just the sort of surge state that can
give people the strength of ten ordinary beings in a life-or-death crisis.
One of the more powerful nurses literally sat on Lokeman in bed; he
wrapped the patient in "a WWF hold," as Chase saw it, and still he was
being tossed and bucked as easily as a child. Meanwhile Takahashi and
Chase worked to get restraints around Lokeman's chest.

Even this might not work for long, for Lokeman would kill himself
with his exertions. He had been given benzodiazepines earlier for his
seizures, the same tranquilizing drugs given to patients suffering from
anxiety. But they were plainly having a so-called paradoxical effect, increasing the bursts of adrenaline and its cousins to intensify his brute
strength against those his brain said were trying to kill him. He fought
for his life, and that would soon prove fatal.

Monitors screamed. Lokeman's blood pressure was dropping at the
moment his brain most needed blood. His lab tests were horrifying: everywhere, he was septic, suffering infections of everything from Hepatitis
C, probably another drug-abuse result, to microbial invasions. Chase called
Anish Bhardwaj upstairs in his office. He was the attending who would be
on call all night, her unseen shadow, either in his office or at home.
Lokeman was already on a vasopressor—a drug that would raise his low

blood pressure by constricting his arteries. With Bhardwaj's okay, she took step one, giving Lokeman a large dose of a second pressor. Such drugs, of course, could send a person's blood-vessel pressure from low—or hypotensive—to high—or hypertensive. Lokeman could die of a heart attack. Or increased blood pressure to give the brain needed oxygen could lead to a vessel's rupture and thus a brain hemorrhage. Every step she might take to save him from one fate would put him in the path of another.

She called the trauma team chief who had treated Lokeman on his admission a day earlier. The surgeon immediately asked why Chase had not inserted a Swann-Ganz catheter to measure Lokeman's pulmonary artery pressure, the surest, quickest way to track erratic blood pressure. Another quick call to Bhardwaj: "Help." She had never inserted a Swann-Ganz. "Don't worry about it," Bhardwaj said. "What would a Swann-Ganz tell us that we don't already know? His pressure is through the floor. We need to get it up."

Having given Lokeman the second pressor Chase could do nothing but wait, and in crisis, you never want to wait. She headed for the waiting room, where Lokeman's large family had gathered, to tell them things were not going well. But, anticipating a hard night now, she knew that repeating this long trip to the waiting room at every crisis would not work. She had eight other patients in critical care, each needing his or her share of attention and response if the nurse on duty should call. She had a hard, angry spot in her heart for the idea of telling a family at one moment that all was okay, and, on the next trip down that long corridor so far from the NICU, that its son and brother was dead. She had to keep them informed minute by minute.

When she was in high school, her grandmother had had open-heart surgery. Chere and her mother waited for the surgeon to bring them word, and when he finally appeared he was cold and curt. The patient was doing as well as could be expected. When they pressed him with questions, he said there was nothing more to tell and walked out. They were terrified. Did that mean near death or doing well? She would never do that. Nothing was as bad as not knowing.

In the waiting room sat Jay's mother, Ardelia, and his siblings, Joey, Cathy and Vernon Reid, plus several of their children and other relatives. But there was an unused patient room in the Neuro ICU, and she decided to bring the family in, right next to Jay, so she could post them minute-by-minute in what might be a fatal night. "We need enough chairs for everyone," she told Takahashi, and between them they set up a seating circle in the empty room, so they could witness the entire crisis. Risky business, allowing the family to watch these traumatic events up close, without training or preparation, but, she decided, worth the risk.

The news only got worse. The added pressor did nothing; Lokeman's blood pressure continued to drop. Now his blood labs showed acidosis— acidic blood—the sign that his brain, liver, kidneys, every organ including the heart itself, were not getting enough oxygen. In addition to being a signal that tissues were being destroyed, the acidity was dangerous in itself. She paged Bhardwaj, now at home, and with his okay added a third pressor, this one working to boost Lokeman's blood pressure in a different way.

No go. Worse, newly agitated, he raged again. By 10 p.m., Chase was literally stretched across his chest, her face pressed in his, pleading: "Stop fighting me! I'm trying to help you! Stop fighting me!"

And suddenly, to that insistent but never angry voice, he responded, quieting.

But now his kidneys and liver were failing from acidosis. Each time she looked at the lab report, his numbers were worse. And, as she knew was inevitable, soon after that, Lokeman's kidneys simply stopped working. This could be the end, Chase thought. She ordered the dialysis machine, to take over for Lokeman's kidneys, in the faint hope that they would come to life again. But the acidosis was still climbing; it would kill brain cells and perhaps even sooner lead to cardiac arrest. She gave him bicarbonate of soda, the same base that neutralizes stomach acid against indigestion, pumped directly into his blood.

In five hours, 18 liters of very salty water were pumped through Lokeman's arteries, to suck water out of his brain and keep the inevitable fluid buildup from destroying cerebral tissue with pressure.

Still his pressure dropped. Again Takahashi was on the phone from down the hall: He's agitated again! And again Chase was on his chest, repeating, "Stop fighting me! I'm trying to help you. Please stop fighting me." Restoring calm. But not blood pressure, not kidneys, certainly not consciousness.

On the phone to Bhardwaj: "We've added a third pressor. No one's ever on more than two pressors. What am I doing wrong?"

"You're not doing anything wrong," came the reply. "Sometimes patients die, Chere. You are doing all you can. Maybe he is supposed to die."

And finally came the wee hours of the morning, when every doctor on call prays for 7 a.m. and the beginning of morning rounds. The cavalry riding in. Support, company, relief at the beleaguered outpost. But this was Sunday morning, so rounds would begin two hours late, at 9 a.m. How to hang on? .

In the quiet, at last, she was able to look backward and forward. She was finished. He was finished. To the Lokemans she says: "I don't think Jay will make it. I think he is going to die." Now she began losing it, though she tried to hang on to her composure. "I'm losing. We're losing. I'm fighting as hard as I can, every way I know. And I'm losing."

Suddenly, startling her, the entire family jumped up and surrounded her, hugging her. "It's all right," she heard, over and over. "We've been watching. You have done everything you can. If he dies, it's what God means for him." Over and over: "It's in God's hands. You've done all you can do." And this from his mother, brothers, sister.

The words calmed her, then gave her a new burst of energy; but they gave her no new insights. Bhardwaj was right, there *were* no new insights. There was nothing left. She poured in more bicarbonate of soda, and that alone could give Lokeman cardiac arrest.

She called Bhardwaj again. "Listen, Chere," he said. "This guy is sick and he's going to die. This happens. He's ready to die. Let him go. There is nothing left for you to do."

"So I shouldn't call you."

"Call me as often as you like," he said. "I just won't have anything new to tell you, because there is nothing more to tell you. But keep calling me."

To Holli Takahashi she cried, "Anish says we should give up. I can't give up." And Takahashi: "If you say quit, I'll quit. If you push on, I'll push on."

Nothing worked. Lokeman's pH level continued to drop, indicating increasing blood acid. She added a fourth pressor, which, she knew, made absolutely no sense medically. She was doing this simply to do something, and that was a very bad reason to do something in an emergency.

As she stood at Lokeman's bed at 7:30 a.m., Anish suddenly appeared at her side, 90 minutes early, though she would learn this was usual for him. "This guy doesn't look nearly as sick as I expected," Bhardwaj said.

"I don't know what got him to this point," she said. "But it wasn't me. And I sure don't know what's next."

She had been concerned about giving Lokeman any more bicarb. Bhardwaj tripled it. She had exhausted the pressors and then some.

Bhardwaj dropped two but added what seemed to her a huge dose of the drug Levophed, which residency wags had termed "Leave 'em dead." So powerful was this pressor's action as a blood vessel constrictor that it often literally clamped down the circulation in the limbs, forcing increased blood pressure centrally, to the viscera and brain. But the nickname, Bhardwaj knew, was an exaggeration; recent studies had indicated Levophed was safe when used correctly.

Within an hour, Lokeman was out of crisis. Whether by act of God, four pressors, or Leave 'em dead, he lay on dialysis, full of infection, though out of status epilepticus—a sick, sick man, but alive for now.

Chase has reflected back on her grandmother's cold-hearted cardiac surgeon, a man her grandmother, as a private-duty nurse, came to know as a friend. He had been mortified when reminded of his behavior to Chere and her mother that day of surgery. "The unit was full of my patients," he had said. "And every one was trying to die. No matter what I did, all my patients were trying to die." Perhaps that was why he had not been willing to speak to them; perhaps his anger and frustration had just shut him down.

Chase had never seen a patient try as hard to die as Lokeman had, "him with both feet in the grave and me pulling as hard as I could." But then, when she had done everything she could, he had hung on, then came back a bit, not because of her.

Lokeman's story might end here and now, family at his side, loving him after all, putting all the responsibility right on him yet forgiving him to begin again. Cathy Reid brought in fellow church members, whom she remembers being joined every day by hospital staff, to pray for her brother. But for a life story, the only ending that is a given is the one Chase had just averted.

CHAPTER 4

Bottom of the Night

A S ANISH BHARDWAJ had prepared to leave that Saturday evening, he did not share Chere Chase's optimism about Jay Lokeman's prospects. It was not that he foresaw trouble. Too much was going on with Lokeman that he did not understand, having nothing to do with the grave status epilepticus. After Bhardwaj had triaged Lokeman the night before, they had gotten him stabilized almost as soon as he came into the unit, but by Saturday evening he was alternately agitated and comatose, and his blood pressure was erratic. Cause: idiopathic, a very unpleasant word. A pathology of unknown origin. A potential killer in the dark. Lokeman's swollen, pink, mottled skin was a sign of possible necrotizing fasciitis, the so-called "flesh-eating bacteria." All signs pointed to virulent invaders—bacterial, viral or both, in addition to the hepatitis C he certainly had.

After turning Lokeman over to Chase, Bhardwaj ran up the long flight to the eighth floor, to the neurointensive care division and into his office next to Mirski's. The codirector's office was far smaller; but, in terms of working space, there was not much difference. Still, the offices reflected their owners' characters and positions, as well as the very different dynamics of their daily routines as academic clinicians. The office through which Mirski passed, the center of gravity in his endless daily perambulation, was neat as a pin; desks, conference table were all cleared of paperwork. Bhardwaj's horizontal surfaces were stacked with research results, manuscripts in preparation or that he was reviewing for journals, article reprints for reference. If Mirski's two obsessions are work and family, Bhardwaj's are work and work. Research and doctoring, lab and Neuro ICU. Dr. Anish, as he calls himself for simplicity in the unit, arrives at the hospital between 4 and 4:30 a.m., though he admits to running a bit later on weekends. He leaves in the evening. "Work, work, work!" Ski Lower says of him, rolling her eyes. "That's all Anish does. I have told him and told him, 'Anish, you have a wife. It's late. Go home to your wife.' But does he listen?"

Bhardwaj's wife, Izumi Harukuni, is a resident in anesthesia, so when he does go home, of course, she is often on call. They are an increasingly common medical family: the two-doctor household with both on the run. Izumi was a board-certified attending anesthesiologist in Japan. She came to Johns Hopkins to do research and, by chance, was teamed in the lab with Anish. During two years working side by side, they fell in love and married, and, as all foreign-trained physicians must, she then began her residency training all over again, from internship onward.

Bhardwaj's office has room for two guest chairs. The desk light sends a bright cone outward from the focus, enough to illuminate the aphorisms printed via computer that look down from the walls. If the stacks of papers give away his research interests, this writing on the wall offers a prospect of his inspirations:

"Every day, try to help someone who cannot reciprocate your kindness."

"May our adversities make us strong."

"Courage is not defined by those who fought and did not fall."

And these on achievement:

"The importance of winning is not what we get for it, but what we become because of it."

"No victory is worth the sacrifice of ideals."

And finally, "Where you find success, there you find sacrifice."

Bhardwaj hails from South Africa, where his father was an engineer on some of the African continent's major skyscrapers. After medical school in South Africa, he came to New York for residency training in neurology, at Mount Sinai Hospital.

The room's only illumination day or night comes from the pearl, diffuse light through the door opposite the desk at the south end and the bright cone flooding the desk and its content, the kind of light from which Rembrandt figures emerge. Emerging is a dark-complected, thoughtful face. Of somewhat short stature, he commonly walks with both hands in white-coat pockets, balling them deep, when deep in thought.

He was still in his office when his pager screeched on Saturday night—Chere's first call. Because of Lokeman's low and still dropping blood pressure, she wanted to add a second vasopressor. The drug would constrict Lokeman's arteries and thus increase the pressure of the blood that would reach his brain and other vital organs. The idea is the same as closing down the end of a garden hose with your thumb to push the water higher or farther. With a constant pressure from the source—the pumping heart—the narrower opening will force pressure up at the business end.

Bhardwaj had agreed, headed home, and was off to sleep when the next call came. The trauma surgeon had just asked Chere why she didn't have a Swann-Ganz in Lokeman. "His pressure's dropping and we still don't know why. I've never done a Swann-Ganz."

Bhardwaj had done *many* of them. But inserting a Swann-Ganz catheter is not a benign procedure, in any hands. The balloon-tipped tube is inserted into the pulmonary artery as it heads into the lungs after leaving the heart. The only artery that carries oxygen-depleted blood, it is now making the vital pass through the lungs to reoxygenate. At this critical juncture, the catheter's balloon is briefly inflated and the pressure of the blood-surge against the balloon is measured. It is the most accurate means of gauging blood pressure at one of the most important sites. But it is also possible to rupture the pulmonary artery, in that moment losing the patient.

Though only 40, Anish often reflected that as he got older, or perhaps more experienced, he was not so quick to jump to procedures. The younger doctors always wanted to fix things. He more frequently saw the virtue of *Primum, non nocere:* First, do no harm. Years earlier, the young resident Dr. Bhardwaj visited here as a fellow in October, interviewing for one of the neurointensive openings for the following July. At 5 p.m., to his shock, NICU director Dan Hanley had shaken his hand and said, "Call if there's a problem." "I literally didn't know where the men's room was," he recalls. Still, trial by fire was the traditional way in medicine, and as someone trained under the British system in South Africa, Bhardwaj was no stranger to that regimen.

Problem? In the middle of the night, Mrs. H____, suffering from leukemia *and* myasthenia gravis, a sometimes-fatal nerve disease, had been brought into the unit postop. She needed reinsertion of her central line—

the catheter that reads oxygen-depleted venous blood as it enters the heart through the superior vena cava. Bhardwaj might have been a senior resident at Mount Sinai, but here he was just a visiting fellow. He was in charge. He inserted the Swann-Ganz line and instantly punctured Mrs. H____'s pleural membrane. This critical sac holds a slight vacuum so that the lungs can reinflate after they exhale. One lung immediately collapsed. In a flash Bhardwaj was on the phone to Hanley, his attending. "Call cardio," Hanley said. "They'll take care of it. And don't worry about it."

Mrs. H____ recovered without a hitch. Bhardwaj had just brought about the most common iatrogenic—that is, treatment-induced—morbidity in intensive care. It was called "dropping a lung," or, correctly but less colorfully, causing a pneumothorax, and in his turn he had had to comfort and support many a resident in similar straits. Also in his turn he had become more cautious about leaping to the invasive procedure, even when motives were the best.

The next morning, Hanley had been supportive and kind. But more important, in the coming years, he led Bhardwaj through the subtler sides of medicine, the art of it that borders on mystique. Many times, leaving a patient's room during a period of calm recovery, during his fellowship years, Hanley had turned to Bhardwaj and said in so many words: "Better watch this patient, Anish. In 48 hours he's going to be in trouble." And so he would be. Science had been the first overpowering draw of neurointensive care for Bhardwaj. The final, irresistible lure was this uncanny part that took years to grasp but was never fully learned.

NOW, FROM HOME, he was asking Chere Chase: "What would a Swann-Ganz catheter tell us about this patient that we don't already know?" And they discussed the actions Chere was deliberating, Bhardwaj weighing in as needed. She was a graduate neurologist and knew what she was about. Once arrived at and agreed to, the decisions the fellows made needed to be carried out by them alone. Already on two pressors, Lokeman would be boosted to three. Bhardwaj passed on thoughts about what side effects or co-events to lost blood pressure she ought to look out for, and they talked about his antibiotics for the infection that was raging inside him.

At some hour in the middle of the night, as Lokeman's crisis deepened, Chase's page found Bhardwaj back at his desk on the eighth floor, head bent to the research piled at his side and in his computer. That research so intimately relates to what happens one floor below that for him there is no separating them. The aim of such research is to go "from bench to bedside." New discoveries—of how things work or don't, of tools, of protocols—must be moved swiftly from the research bench to the patient's bedside. Every clinician-researcher dreams of making a fundamental discovery—"Eureka!"—and seeing it realized in a new standard of patient care. Exciting stuff. And rare.

Naturally, the nuts and bolts can be mind-numbing. Apply for grants. If successful—increasingly uncommon over the years—carry out the meticulous work for months or years. Analyze data gathered by you and the assistants and technicians supported by the grants. Write up the work and send it out for review and hoped-for publication. Respond to criticism and resubmit. Present your data at conferences before and after publication. Write reports justifying grants awarded, and, completing the circle, apply for new grants to fuel the next round of research you hope will answer a few of the questions burning a hole in your brain.

The spur? Certainly not the lure of gold. There is no wealth to be had in this. At Johns Hopkins, as at nearly all major research hospitals, faculty are paid a fixed salary. They see no personal financial gain from the grants they win, but to survive and be promoted, win grants they must. Some, like Bhardwaj, express contempt for wealth that would startle the average patient. "Medicine and money do not mix," he says with quiet fervor. Is fame the spur? Among peers, perhaps, but few ever make discoveries over the course of a lifetime that the rest of us hear of. There is, to be sure, the pride of association: they are professors in Johns Hopkins Medicine. That's cachet, all right, but is it enough to fuel this kind of drive? Maybe it's obsessive curiosity, or the desire to do good, or, maybe, as in so many arenas, there's little that can be generalized except what is obvious: they all seem to love what they do.

Still, of all the people of this story, Bhardwaj perhaps is closest to the paradigm of the Johns Hopkins researcher-clinician, the academic doctor who skimps on neither side, driven by polar forces from one toward the other and back again. This Saturday morning, as always, his desk holds pieces of each phase of several grants and applications on which his name appears as principal investigator—the honcho—or as a co-investigator. The work displays his many interests. Brain edema, excitotoxicity, stroke, hemorrhage. But all his interests dance around this common question: Why do brain cells die? To ask such a question, you must either be very naive or very savvy, deep in the problem. For example, a quarter century ago, scientists asked, "What causes cancer?" They were not looking toward the ever-expanding list of carcinogens. They were looking for a few common mechanisms by which the carcinogens did their damage, in hopes of finding a few common solutions. They're still looking, but they have found some, by looking down the track of cancer genes and the many ways they are activated and turned off. Like that quest, this one also begins with the understanding that there are almost countless ways brain cells can be assaulted. But do these assaults likewise funnel down to a few common events at the edge of death? If so, how might those events be prevented?

When some of the neurons in a circuit in a patient's brain fire out of control, in seizure, they occasionally recruit others, to become generalized. Whether of one focus or generalized, seizures can form feedback loops to create status epilepticus, like Jay Lokeman's. Uncontrolled, that excitation kills the neurons en masse. Now here is an apparently different path to death: when someone's brain is deprived of blood for any reason— say, from a stroke—the downstream neurons die of oxygen-deprivation. And another: a brain on the edge of death often swells, and it is not merely because water is puffing up the matrix between the cells; the neurons themselves are bloated with water. What do these three things—excitotoxicity, stroke infarction, edema—have in common? What processes do all these cells go through in their death throes? Bhardwaj and others are finding that in fact startling similarities in the death mechanisms underlie these very different brain cell killers.

Follow this path a while. Start with "excited to death," the result of excitotoxicity. The neuron's job is to fire. Or not. That's it for for the neuron as computer bit. Which one it does at any given moment results from a simple computation. Sum up the neuron's incoming orders from other neurons on the positive side—fire—and the negative—don't fire. The larger number wins, all or nothing. The excitatory or inhibitory message is sent by means of a chemical messenger called a neurotransmitter.

The most common excitatory neurotransmitter in the brain is glutamate, and that's interesting because this amino acid is also one of the ordinary building blocks of proteins, and, in slightly modified form, it is one of the best known to the average person. One part sodium and one part chloride yields table salt. One part sodium and one part glutamate yields monosodium glutamate, MSG, the often-troublesome "seasoning salt" found in some meat tenderizers and restaurant recipes. Here's an obvious problem for the brain. Glutamate, the building block, must be available in huge quantities throughout the body. Glutamate, the excitatory and, therefore, dangerous neurotransmitter must be available only in very tiny, very tightly controlled quantities. The brain's solution is to lock up glutamate on its side of the blood-brain barrier in tight compartments whose locks are powered by oxygen, shipped in the body's major energy fuel cell, ATP.

What happens, then, when an ischemic stroke or hemorrhage cuts off the oxygen supply to part of the brain? ATP dwindles and the locks fall open. Glutamate rushes out of storage, flooding the spaces between neurons and, with oxygen radicals that might be imagined as particles sparking like downed transmission wires, begins destroying the neurons. Excitotoxicity. Same death as status epilepticus, different starting points.

One of Bhardwaj's research projects aims to counter the rush of glutamate precisely where its overactive messaging is causing neuronal death, while not disturbing its crucial work throughout the rest of the trillion brain cell universe.

Continue along the path to edema, another cause of cell death. The fire/don't fire electrical pulse of the brain cell can be seen in a chorus of millions, as waves on an electroencephalogram, or EEG. To maintain the electrical potential needed for appropriate pulsing, the brain cell uses a pump that forces potassium into the cell and sodium out. The pump needs a lot of energy to do so and gets it, again, from the body's major fuel cell molecule, ATP. Deprive the cell of oxygen, and ATP dwindles and the sodium-potassium pump falls still. The cell can no longer fire when needed. And worse in the long run, sodium rushes into the cell and does what it does in any brine solution. It makes the cell bloat with water, in this case often until it explodes. Edema. Cause: loss of that same ATP.

SCREECH. THE PAGER: Lokeman was still sinking—crashing was more like it—through the long night. The only surprise is that he had not reached bottom and died. Chere had decided, based on Lokeman's numbers, to add yet a third vasopressor drug in an effort to boost his blood pressure. They talked back and forth a few minutes. Bhardwaj approved, especially the course of saline solution to keep swelling down in Lokeman's brain. To her concerns that she had failed to do something important, he reassured her, "You're not doing anything wrong." A pause, then the solemn caution against letting herself take this too personally: "Sometimes patients are just supposed to die, Chere. You are doing all you can." No God or destiny invoked here, just the idea that much of healing or failing to heal lies outside medicine. "Maybe he is supposed to die."

"Sometimes I get depressed," Bhardwaj said in his office, long after that night. "So much in medicine *cannot* be done. You do all you can do and people die." And then comes the far more difficult question in taking "heroic measures" to "save" a brain-wrecked person. What is he being saved *for*? Will he recover, or will he rise only to some dim level of unawareness where he will persist for months or years, vegetative?

Chere Chase had the training—the years of resident's call and the year as chief resident. She had impeccable skills, or she would not be here. Nevertheless, there was, in the moment of taking charge, real terror. There had to be. There was the fear of death, and the heart-wrenching fear that you might cause it. You realized that, indeed, this was up to you. Two years from now, Bhardwaj knew, she might decide to take the next step, shouldering the the whole unit, its operation and the lives of every last patient. She would be an attending. There would be no one to call. There would be consultation from other specialists if need be, but she would be the one leaned on.

Back down he went to the gateway of his research—literally and figuratively—the blood-brain barrier. In the energy processes of the brain, just two molecules stand as the fundament in every sequence of events. Glucose and oxygen, the fuel and its partner, are the constant passengers through this labyrinthine membrane linking blood vessels and brain. Many molecules are stored in the brain for use as needed. Not these two. They must be delivered as needed by the blood. Their functions? Release of energy, and control of the release of energy. What could be simpler or more complex?

As he works on these problems through the night, Bhardwaj is living at the sub-microscopic level, where the single neuron's many kinds of channels port molecules in and out with smooth, precise control. The neuron is a gargantuan space station with different kinds and levels of access controls swirling over a vast, complex territory, a living world unto itself. A world where a systematic breakdown—not the failure of one pump or one gate but of all of one kind—can lead to explosion or the frozen silence of death.

Try to make a simple model of what was going on here over that Saturday night, to get a feel for the whole. Start with the Meyer Building, these two floors, seven and eight; ignore Bhardwaj's drive home and back. If you were to make a 3D map, a complex schema that would locate each of these two players—Chase and Bhardwaj—not merely physically but in the story, putting Anish Bhardwaj in this puzzle is far more difficult than locating Chase. Chase is moving like a shot, but you can watch her through the night and her motions tell the story so simply that no TV watcher would need sound to understand. Each motion is purposeful, pragmatic. Even those carried out in desperation—or especially those—all aim to hang onto Jay Lokeman, and as she said so well, to drag him back. Inside her head or outside, now watching the monitors of an elderly stroke patient, prescribing, or taking a page from Holli Takahashi to rush back to Lokeman's bed, or stopping to discuss what might be final matters with Ardelia and her children: She is being a doctor, and this is what doctors do.

Bhardwaj sits. For most of his waking hours this night he barely moves and when he does it's a distraction from the research. Yet he moves up and down the universe. This is not to exalt these activites. He is *doing* the same things we all do when we sit and work our brains. This difficulty in the telling—What is he *doing?*—has nothing to do with Bhardwaj in particular, but with our brains and what they're up to. And they're always up to something. On the phone to Chere Chase, he has placed himself in the unit, at her side, to see what she sees, without moving. (Mirski: "On your boards, don't try to sit and think what you'd do." *Put yourself here. See.*) Bhardwaj sees Lokeman's chart, the numbers stable or plunging, with the same inner eye that would be working the numbers if he were one floor down—ten or so feet—from where he sits. And a trice later, he has hung up the phone and is back in a world of neuronal networks, excitotoxicity, failed pumps too tiny ever to see, beyond anything that we call vision—except metaphorically. And it's all just two orders of magnitude down from here. Imagine that, in coming up one level of stairs, he had climbed not 10 or 15 feet, but to a macroscopic level ten times larger than the one he'd left, and that another flight would put him 100 times larger, and another flight 1000 times. Six flights up to a million-fold increase in macro-scale, a player among the stars. Six flights down to a million-fold decrease into micro-scale, swimming among giant cells in a world measured in microns instead of meters, and down from there.

Bhardwaj's mind rises to the NICU, then plunges down some other kind of stairwell, down orders of magnitude to the levels at which these things are caused. Running stairs. This is how they all train. But it is not different in kind from how anyone *trains.* Jay Lokeman's problems started at eye-level, street-level, cruising for drugs, doing them, fighting, crashing. But what continues now, as surely as it has gone on for days, is completely invisible. At eye level, Jay is at one moment deathly still, at the next a raging bull with the power of ten strong men, then as quickly heaving and gasping, weak with plunging blood pressure, and up again. You have to go down orders of magnitude to understand the events. What is going on at some microscopic level that is ending up here in this contradictory, lethal behavior?

Skipping up and down orders of magnitude is no super-power, but it does take discipline to do well and routinely. Training has a lot of commonality. The now-cliché coach tells his players kneeling in group solidarity that only "total 110 percent concentration will win!" Concentration on what? On winning, the goal, the end in view. Not on the separate steps to get there, nor the separate steps to avoid the obstacles in the path. These it is the function of training to engrain deep in the player's brain, to be pulled together at will, to entrain by will.

"Get me some *will* neurons." There aren't any, but there are small, linked networks of neurons whose loss would rob your will, pure and simple. Harmony, synergy, all the forces harnessed by the hauling together of separate motions toward one end. The force of total concentration we admire in the pitcher, violinist, high diver is perhaps at one apotheosis in the neurosurgeon, whose motions are small and steady, ever smaller and ever steadier, whose every motion and concentration is brought to bear on one tiny place, tiny problem, unbelievably narrow range of error.

But that is not the neurointensivist. The approach is wholly different. No matter what the problem that brought a patient into the NICU, intensivists must make rolling diagnoses, thinking on their feet, immediately responding. This is what neurointensivists say repeatedly. They must be concerned with the whole patient. Readiness to focus, and to draw back and refocus, is the unending demand for the intensivist.

Case in point. Here is Jay Lokeman, brought into the Neurointensive Care Unit for only one reason, and that one of the deadliest—status epilepticus. But, presto, that isn't even a factor in his night-long momentum toward death. The lesson has nothing immediately to do with excitotoxicity or edema. *His blood pressure is falling,* the immediate consequence being that his brain is being starved and will become ischemic, just as it would in stroke. Then he will have a fatal reason for being in this unit, related to both excitotoxicity and edema. Keep your eye on the problem, but not too closely. Quick as a wink, it's not the problem, blood pressure is. Or is it renal failure that will kill him? Or sepsis?

It was morning, Bhardwaj saw, as he slipped out of his office to see how things were going in the unit. He headed down the single flight and punched the large button to swing open the Neuro ICU doors. Chase was still there by Lokeman's bed. Quiet as stone. Blood pressure very low but stable. Status epilepticus under control, for now. On dialysis. No kidneys now, or maybe ever. Hepatitis C. Septic as hell. "This guy doesn't look nearly as sick as I expected," he told her.

CHAPTER 5

Fire and Flood

April is the cruellest month, breeding
Lilacs out of the dead land, mixing
Memory and desire, stirring
Dull roots with spring rain.

SOMEWHERE IN T. S. Eliot's brain April was woven, and he sent it along to the rest of us, where it emerges from a billion tendrils bound up as consciousness, one chord struck out of that many notes. When it comes, it either seduces as promised, or it arrives like the thinnest veneer over a wasteland, paint on a wreckage. This is not April, the calendar month. The calendar is stuck on July, 2001. It will take a while to see where and when April insinuates itself.

We hover above Long Island, New York, a long, skinny piece of territory stretching all the way from "the city," where its western tip forms the boroughs of Queens and Brooklyn, to fork nearly 150 miles northeast into the sandy countrysides of Orient Point and Montauk, and sharing yachting waters with Rhode Island. About 2.75 million people live here in hundreds of suburban communities jammed cheek by jowl and joined by networks of arteries sprung out of near-nothing during the baby-boom years, turning crossroads with Indian names and farm markets into the pixels of Megalopolis.

Two families who figure prominently in this story connect at one Long Island town—Huntington— though, as noted at the outset, none of the family members are known to have met. Ambulances carried two of them to Columbia, one of just a few of the highest level neuro centers in this part of the country, delivering them into the Neurological Intensive Care Unit as the patients of Stephan Mayer. There the cases radically diverged. Their events played out in different realms of the brain, with consequences as different as night and day, but sharing this one link in the functioning of the brain, so hard to put in precise word or phrase: the mixing of memory and desire, the annealing of wanting and planning, thinking and feeling, of hard lines of logic and the color eruptions of emotion.

FIRST THERE ARE THE BECKS, Joe and Gail, just into their thirties with two small boys and a mortgage, *familia americana* at the end of the millennium. Joe is a dark-haired, husky man of middle height with a ready smile and outgoing personality, a yarn spinner, a dreamer who has worked with some success to make it as a writer who still loves his work as a high school English teacher. Gail is quieter, more appraising, but with a great sense of humor and a smile that lights Joe up more than a decade after they met, nearly ten years into their marriage. Like most close couples, they are a study in both contrasts and unions. She was born and raised in Hicksville, 20 miles from their current home in Huntington

Station. Her parents, Herb and Susan Domroe, still live in Hicksville and both Becks are close to them. Like many, Gail majored in English. Like some, she truly loved its literature—especially *Hamlet*—and loves it still. But Joe is the writer; she is the editor. She has spent the last several years as a technical editor for the American Institute of Physics, in nearby Melville, and since Ian was born has worked at home. Joe is adventuresome, one of six kids and a Navy brat, born in Pensacola and growing up in port cities from Yokohama to Monterey. He finally finished high school in Huntington. He had begged Gail to go with him on photo safari through the Serengeti with his fellow anthropology students at the State University of New York at Oneonta, but she was and is a homebody and still has never left the country.

Joe and Gail share a two-level duplex home with Gail's sister and brother-in-law, Rachel and John Kinsella, and their two kids. They share baby-sitting duties, and the four children are never at a loss for playmates.

The Becks are old enough to have settled into family life, young enough to hold the memory of their first meeting in close reach. Joe opened the door of his dorm room to see "the most beautful, brown-eyed girl I'd ever set eyes on, her face framed by a long mane of strawberry hair that hung to her wasit." Gail Domroe, 19 on that August 26, had come with her girlfriend to meet up with *her* boyfriend, instead met his roommate, Joe Beck, just out of the shower and clad in nothing but a towel. They married four years later and worked out their different interests in their jobs. But as for Gail and physics, she says about her job choice that it is neither her field nor her hobby. She is a technical editor, minding the style, grammar and sentence structure of articles already peer-reviewed for publication. Joe kicked around: newspaper reporter, trade magazine writer, landscaper. And finally English teacher, at first in Lawrence Middle School, now at Plainview High School.

June. The end of the school year brings a promising flurry of activity for the Becks after what has been a hard time. Only a few weeks earlier, Gail's father, Herb, underwent triple-bypass heart surgery. He is having a difficult recovery, especially troubled by loss of memory. But as summer fills the Long Island beaches and school vacation begins, things look hopeful. The worst appears over. The weekend before, Joe and Gail had taken the boys for a visit with his parents in Southold, near the Island's V-projection northeast into the Atlantic, an hour's drive from home in Huntington Station. There they took Andrew, 6, and Ian, 15 months , to one of the many carnivals that light up the seaside towns in summer.

Andrew was just getting over chicken pox, but he appeared to be fully recovered and enjoyed himself on this outing. The weather was perfect. Nothing was wrong or unusual. They frequently note this because they've been asked so often. They look back and scan their memories for something out of place, a clue. All Joe can remember is that the area around the carnival, like much of Long Island, was sandy, dotted with marsh. Somewhere, almost certainly, the harbinger was there but too small and common to take seriously if seen, heard, even felt. Sometime, likely that weekend but maybe later right here in the house, a mosquito came dancing on the air, one of millions along the East Coast in any summer of any year. A minor irritant. But that won't do. It isn't in us to stop searching for causes that can be firmly located and carefully avoided: Watch for falling rocks. In event of fire, use staircase. Beware mosquitos?

On this Saturday, June 22, the day after school closed, the Becks had been headed for the American Institute of Physics annual picnic, but Gail didn't feel very well. She had been fighting what seemed like flu all week and finally decided she wasn't up to the picnic. Her legs felt like iron. She lay down on the living-room couch and slept most of the day. Joe spent the afternoon at the computer, writing. About four o'clock he heard Gail moan, then nothing. As he rushed into the living room, she moaned loudly again, then began thrashing, then nothing again.

Joe later wrote the next thing he remembers:

> *"Gail, Gail!" The paramedic repeated my wife's name as she worked over her in the ambulance. We were on our way to Huntington Hospital after she had had a major convulsive seizure . . .*
>
> *[The paramedic] shined a light in her eyes. "Gail!" she repeated. "Can you hear me?" She moaned and uttered unintelligibly. . .*
>
> *A string of questions: Prior seizures? Illegal drug use? Smoker?*
>
> *"No." I bent down to hold her hand. "Look, can we just get to the hospital?" Fear and anger welled up in me and my eyes were moist.*
>
> *"We're doing the best we can, sir. We'll be there in about six minutes."*

SO THEY WERE, and the Domroes joined them minutes later. Gail's seizures increased in severity and duration. She did not regain consciousness. The antiseizure drugs she was given dampened but would not quell the seizures, even the powerful barbiturate phenobarbital. Finally, staff neurologist Barbara Allis told them what the doctors knew. Gail was having intractable seizures, "intractable" meaning nothing seemed to relieve them for more than a short period. Seizures had progressed from focal—localized within a particular region—to become generalized throughout her cortex. And instead of slowing under the powerful drugs that dampen neurons' firing out of control, the seizures were worsening.

What was happening? If we could spread the six-layer sheet of the neuronal cortex out and actually see the flashes of seizures as thunderbolts, we would see multiple lightning storms searing its critical regions, more streaks of lightning surging back and forth, seemingly random in their patterns. And like lightning, these seizures would destroy. There would be no flame, but the constant firing eventually would burn out the neurons. The unrelenting bursts would lead to excitotoxicity, whose synergy would combine single harmful effects into lethal combinations just as Gail's single seizures had spread outward.

Day after day, the storms played out. Yet every test over the next five days would prove frustratingly normal. Blood proteins normal. Spinal fluid told that the brain's health appeared normal. Temperature. Blood pressure. No matter what the test, normal—frustrating because seizures broke through every powerful drug, and something causes seizures that is not at all normal.

Gail, who had had several seizures on Saturday, was in full status epilepticus, the seizures coming so frequently that they were for all intents and purposes constant, and life threatening. Some epilepsy patients suffer multiple daily seizures yet have no brain damage years later. Why is status so deadly? Because neurons do not have time to recover, to rebuild their energy stores, between firings. David Treiman, one of the leading investigators of status epilepticus, believes that even two seizures should be considered status if they are close enough together to prevent the firing brain cell from recovering.

Allis recommended transferring Gail to Columbia's NICU. As the neurologist and Joe Beck clambered into the ambulance behind Gail's gurney for the journey down the Long Island Expressway to Columbia, there seemed little if any hope for something like recovery. But there was hope for life, for some kind of life that would have to be invented. That would have to do, Joe decided. Anything would be better than losing Gail. Thank God he had the summer off. They were insured, but how much beyond their coverage would this carry them? The boys were with the Kinsellas now, but he would have to get home soon for them. Gail would not be working. Joe knows this trip on the LIE as any Long Islander would, making a run to the city. There was too much time to think and too few facts to stoke the thinking, so the questions just jumped and danced.

They were in the city now, finally pulling in to the ambulance entrance of Columbia's New York Presbyterian Hospital on Fort Washington Avenue, the George Washington Bridge looming to the north. Finally they'd reached the fourth floor: Neurological Intensive Care Unit.

S T E P H A N M A Y E R L E D afternoon rounds on Thursday, June 27. The year was 1996. This is how he saw Gail Beck just hours after her admission:

Diagnoses: 1. Status epilepticus, 2. Idiopathic encephalopathy possibly secondary to encephalitis . . .

Chief Complaint: 31-year-old woman with status epilepticus . . .

Her brain is practically on fire, Mayer saw, so convulsed in the horrific, non-stop, global brain seizures of status. He had never seen such unremitting, intense seizures, even in status. "Everything in my training, in medicine, neurology, said this woman is a goner. There's nothing to be done," he recalls. Only his readings and experience as an intensivist suggested that extreme treatments might work in the carefully monitored and controlled environment of the NICU. The aggressive approach to status epilepticus championed by Treiman and others was just taking hold in these elite environments. Only a year earlier a case study in the journal *Critical Care Medicine* had described a patient pulled out of status epilepticus after 53 days in "burst suppression," or barbiturate coma. The authors: Marek A. Mirski, Michael A. Williams, Daniel F. Hanley. But few outcomes were as good as theirs, even when patients survived.

The familiar EEG portrays waves dancing in regular patterns throughout the living brain, the music of hundreds of billions of brain cells firing in synchronies so complex that neuroscientists are just beginning to understand them, and they may never do so fully. The patterns displayed on the EEG screen may be modulating bursts fired like timing signals by certain neurons in thousands of networks, to keep the brain in tune, to bind into a single moment dozens of network activities that are occurring in parallel.

But many, if not most, of the firing patterns represent activity that is counterintuitive. The brain in deep sleep is at its most synchronized. Rhythmic pulsings from deep within during sleep appear to *block* transmission of the bursts that communicate sensation and other messages throughout the alert, conscious brain. It's a perfect example of signal jamming.

During a seizure, something crashes chaotically through the harmonies of the brain; however, just as in sleep, this is a well-organized kind of havoc. A wave of lightning replaces the thousands of steady thrums of interconnected networks, and the victim may thrash about wildly or pass out. Another lightning wave may strike, then another. If seizures are not controlled, kindling can occur, just as in a wildfire. In a distant part of the brain, blown as though on the wind by neuronal firings, another local seizure-blaze can break out, and elsewhere another. The metaphors for what happens are vivid, but they remain metaphors: kindling, recruitment, entrainment. But the critical fact about the pathways of seizure is that, unlike an electrical short circuit, neuronal firings are not "jumping their networks." The spread of seizures from local to general follows normal pathways, amplified out of bounds, repeating out of control.

In the worst cases, the separate seizure-fires grow into one firestorm throughout the entire brain, when virtually all the neurons can become involved. That is a generalized seizure, but generalized seizures are usually brief. Any seizures that repeat rapidly represent status epilepticus, and the most serious level of status is generalized. Gail Beck's was the worst case Mayer had ever seen. If he could not stop the firestorm, her brain would burn out—if it had not already—in the metaphorical sense of fatally exhausting itself.

Medications on transfer from Huntington: the anticonvulsant Dilantin and a powerful intravenous drip of the sedative Ativan. But they had failed to stem the explosions. Not even phenobarbital had stopped them. One possibility remained, risky enough that few neurologists outside a neurointensive setting would try it, and that was the barbiturate pentobarbital. A very low dose of sodium pentobarbital provides the so-called truth serum that is a staple of melodrama; a higher dose yields a common general anesthetic. But large doses of the barbiturate hammer the brain's neurons into silence, and, equally dangerously, they drag down the electrical signals that keep the heart beating and can even halt them permanently.

Mayer gave Gail Beck a megadose, suppressing her brain's electrical activity into flatline. The waves vanished from the EEG so it now showed a pattern indistinguishable from that of brain death. The idea was to smother the firings, then slowly bring her back.

After several days Mayer lifted the "barbs." His patient now was in so profound a coma that she registered 3 on the Glasgow Coma Scale, the worldwide quick test of brain function. She could have scored a maximum of 5 in each of three series of tests of responsiveness, for a total GCS of 15. But there is no zero score; 1 is the lowest in each series, a limit brain doctors say is there to remind them that no simple test can be certain. Thus, a cadaver scores 3 on the GCS. As the grim joke goes, on this test you get three points just for showing up. There she was.

Yet even at that level, as Mayer relieved the grip of pentobarbital, the firestorm in Gail's brain resumed, and he pushed her down again. And again. Over days and then weeks she remained in flatline, a state from which many physicians said she could not return. Not at all, never mind to anywhere near "baseline"—that prosaic term for all the rich complexity of life in the moment before.

ENCEPHALITIS WAS the culprit, Mayer was certain, inflammation of the brain that causes swelling and often leads to seizures. The several varieties of encephalitis are caused by viruses, in the United States most commonly carried by mosquitos. Three years later, a new and even deadlier variety would turn up in New York under the name West Nile Virus. Was this, in fact, West Nile itself, years ahead of its emergence? Could have been, but the point is moot. No sign of the cause of Gail's encephalitis had been found, nor would it ever be, and there was never even a confirming test that encephalitis was present. No proof. Idiopathic: occurring without known cause. Another meaning, even stranger and best not dwelt on: self-originating. How can you make science out of that? Making science out of epilepsy has been one of the great challenges of neurology. To get a sense of this, draw back, as though hovering over it as an island, matching brain structures and actions with names of explorers and investigators. It is surprising how many people's paths cross. It is equally surprising how many "good roads" go nowhere.

At one level, epilepsy seems simple—chronic seizures, sometimes with consciousness altered or lost, sometimes with consciousness not affected at all. It has been known by this name for thousands of years. Yet the study of epilepsy, the attempts to grasp the many causes that funnel down into variations on a theme, is so complex and difficult that the physicians who treat it form one of only two board-certified subspecialties in neurology. The first is child neurology; children's developing brains are different enough in their plasticity and function that treating them requires a different finish to residency. Epileptologists' branch is formally known as neurophysiology. Say *anatomy* and we rightly think of a map, for no matter how complex in the relationships of parts, anatomy is structure, still photos. Physiology is the study of dynamics, the parts in motion and communication, if such terms are precise enough for the welter within the body. Motion there is, of many kinds. The speed of flowing blood can be measured by the same means as the speed of galaxies or submarines. And the moving images on the EEG, the thrashing motions of seizure, all clearly suggest the result of electrical discharge, like grabbing a hot wire.

But nowhere else, even in the brain, are appearances at one level so difficult to relate to the underlying events that cause them as they are in neural electricity. Robert Fisher's name comes up often as you travel the tight, small network of epileptologists who balance the worlds of research and patient care—clinician-investigators. Fisher has spent his life studying the electrochemistry of the brain and is "a real dynamic force in our field," one Columbia epileptologist says. Fisher has studied epilepsy in the laboratory and traced it through the often-difficult lives of patients in his clinic and in the neurointensive care units where status epilepticus brings those it has stricken.

"Be careful not to speak of epilepsy as though it were an electrical disease, or a disease of the brain's electrical functions," he cautions in his Stanford office. "It's so much more complicated than that."

As though electricity were simple. More than 200 years after electric current was generated by a battery and "seen" jerking the leg of a dead frog, establishing its neural presence, you can only get a feel for the physical reality of electicity from specialists, be they quantum physicists, biochemists, electrical engineers or epileptologists. Each will define electricity in terms of its manifestations in their own realm, and, in theory, the laws describing electricity's causes and effects are as translatable as currencies. But what is *it*, other than a way of speaking of particular causes and effects? A flow of charge is the most common denominator, and it appears to work here, in the firing of one neuron. But the actual communication between neurons that sets up the "waves" of the EEG is via neurotransmitter molecules that lock into receptors, like keys slipping into and turning locks. Hence the *chemistry* of electrochemistry. In this respect, to speak of the brain as "electric" is like calling the Long Island Railroad an electrical network, rather than a network of steel trains powered by electricity.

Fisher's point is that the convenient electrical analogies break down when you try to employ them in healing the brain. Seizures represent out-of-control firing—measurable electrical pulsing—of masses of neurons, *but the neurons are only out of normal controls.* In fact, the problem is that they are under some other controls. The spiking neurons are very much in alignment, as coordinated as an army marching in perfect step. They are entrained, lined up, but inappropriately. It is difficult to know whether they get that way because their firing mechanisms are too energized or because the inhibitions—the "Don't fire!" signals—are lost. But most investigators these days believe that focal seizures are caused by loss of inhibition. That loss allows normal firing patterns to form a closed loop, as noise can feed back from a bandstand speaker through a microphone and amplifier, then out through the speaker into the mike, leading to an ear-splitting screech. That screech is limited by the power of the components, and in what seems a perfect analogy, most seizures are self-limiting. But there—Fisher's point again—the analogy breaks down. It is now believed that seizures don't stop because the neurons are exhausted of supplies. Exhaustion of supplies leads to brain damage—excitotoxicity—not to the termination of seizures.

Generalized seizures are something else again, and their causes are linked both to structures deep in the brain and to the exquisitely sensitive membrane-skin of neurons.

What causes epilepsy in some people and not in others? Genetics plays a clear role in some childhood epilepsies that run in families, and very recently a faulty gene was found in one of the inherited forms. The inflammation of brain cells through infection, the apparent cause in Gail Beck's case, or because those delicate outer membranes have been bathed in blood, as in a hemorrhage, are other known ways that firing inhibition can be lost and the entrainment can begin in which, like too many soldiers marching in step across a bridge, a destructive rhythm begins and amplifies itself.

Finally, though, to someone who has stared as long and hard at the many faces of epilepsy as Fisher has, another answer suggests itself: Maybe we're all susceptible to seizures, some people only more so. "If we all live long enough, maybe we'll all have a seizure," Fisher hypothesizes. "One person's mean time between seizures is two weeks, maybe mine is 150 years. At some later age, I have one single seizure—not so unusual for anyone, especially as we get older—and I never have another one. I had the first one earlier than my 150 years but won't live long enough for another."

Fisher points out that many of history's leading figures suffered from epilepsy, and it was frequently associated with a possession, holy or demonic. Socrates and St. Paul, Julius Caesar and Joan of Arc, Dostoyevsky, Tchaikovsky, Alexander and Napoleon, James Madison, Vincent Van Gogh—all had epilepsy. Did they have anything else in common? Not apparently. So different are the expressions of epilepsy—it is, after all, a chronic set of symptoms called seizure, with any number of potential underlying causes—that it has taken until the last few decades for specialists to come up with an internationally agreed upon terminology for its many modes.

Does the person lose or change consciousness? If not, it is a simple seizure; if so, it is complex. Does the seizure occur in only one place, emanating from one small spot, its spread limited to a tight, local network of cells? Then it is focal. Does it spread from that single focus to a few other tight, local networks, maybe to its complementary networks on the other side of the brain? Then it is multifocal. On the other hand, if a seizure begins in one place and then spreads throughout the entire cortex, it is termed secondarily generalized. But what if it begins virtually everywhere at once, across most of the vast territory of the cortex? Then it is general— primary generalized.

Interestingly, as noted, those seizures that begin in one place then spread to many, or even become secondarily generalized, follow the paths of normal cortex networks. That is, they don't represent the kind of short circuit in which firing spreads randomly. So far, so good. But the spread throughout cortical pathways doesn't hold for so-called primary generalized seizures. They begin everywhere at once.

How can a seizure literally begin all over the brain at the same moment? Here is yet another doorway into the deepest unknowns of brain function: by emanating from a structure deep within the brain, a structure that sends its firing axons everywhere within the cortex, modulating, relaying, perhaps helping bind sensation, thought, motive and movement into one.

Most of the neurons—the "thinking cells" of the brain—interweave their tendrils among the six layers of the cortex, the deep-folded surface of the brain. But deeper in the brain are other neuronal structures that in lower animals may constitute most of what they've got for a brain. If all the lights in a skyscraper began flickering at once, you would look for a single damaged input source. When firing begins all over the brain at once, you look for someplace like the thalamus. Thalamus and hypothalamus compose the diencephalon, sitting like a metropolis on the giant trade routes between the brain stem—sensation in, action out, rudimentary controls—and the upper brain, the domain of "I." As we'll see, the thalamus has two opposing sets of behaviors that point to it as a major player in those most serious seizures.

In contrast, what would be a likely source for purely *local* out-of-control firing? That is, what parts of the brain normally have to be firing a lot, just to keep us going? Loss of control in these areas, loss of inhibition, would hit harder and faster. The structure twinned in the left and right sides of the brain, called the hippocampus, is the crucial site for laying down new memories—that is, learning—and for recalling what we've learned, or remembering. Long term, the memories are stored throughout our brains. Getting them there requires action within the hippocampus. For all our lives—as long as we can learn a new phone number, remember a new name, see something we've never seen before and embrace or flee from it, then call it all back later on—the hippocampus is a tightly controlled storm of activity. It is the most common site of seizures. Both hippocampi can be damaged by repeated seizures, loss of oxygen in a heart attack, cardiac arrest or near drowning, or through the inflammation of encephalitis. The most common casualties of the damage are learning and memory. The hippocampus is nested within the temporal lobe, which also contains a region involved in language understanding, another hotspot of brain activity. Damage the hippocampus, especially on the left side for most people, and problems in understanding language can occur.

How does brain trauma bring on seizure, even if no hemorrhage is involved? In trauma, neurons are often destroyed, their connections lost, Fisher points out. Even if few new neurons are grown in adults, new connections are made constantly. That is how stroke survivors often regain lost abilities as different structures take over the roles of the missing by forming new pathways. That means, again, furious activity among surrounding neurons, like plants sending roots and spreading into a weeded patch. A frenzy of new growth to a good end—re-learning—but leaving the network more vulnerable to lost control, which the trauma may also engender.

None of this, of course, is status epilepticus. Some years ago, Robert Fisher stood at the bedside of a young woman who had suffered status through a long, painful period. He had brought her out of it with complete success. She lived "two wonderful years," her mother said, and now she had relapsed with no hope of a meaningful recovery. That was at Barrow Neurological Institute in Phoenix, where Fisher was head of neurology and had first call in the Neuro ICU for cases like these. He left Barrow for the endowed professorship he now holds at Stanford. The girl had told her family she wanted meaningful life or none at all, and the family made the decision to follow her wishes and let her go. Fisher did so. Status is special, Fisher says, and perhaps the leading authority on the subject is David Treiman, who coincidentally has just taken over as head of epilepsy at the Barrow Neurological Institute. There, on a dark winter evening when he gets free of his schedule, Treiman elaborates on this mysterious killer. Status epilepticus is called by some a caricature of epilepsy, as though it represented an exaggeration of each of the features that are epilepsy's hallmarks. Epilepsy is common—as many as 1 or even 2 percent of the world's people suffer from it—but status is rare. It can be deadly when generalized, and that is its most common form.

Treiman argues that status epilepticus can be any series of seizures— from the simplest to the most complex, focal or general—marked by lack of recovery of the brain between seizures. That's what causes the damage. The historical figures mentioned suffered epilepsy throughout their lives with no loss of brain function. The damage wrought by status epilepticus, Treiman believes, results from the inability of the neurons to recover before they fire again. That leads to excitotoxicity, but now glutamate, the excitatory neurotransmitter, does not appear to be the major culprit. In status, "there is an alteration in the physiology of the brain such that the normal mechanisms of shutdown fail," Treiman says. *Shutdown* means inhibition.

And that introduces the most common neurotransmitter in the mammalian brain—gamma-aminobutyric acid, mercifully shortened to GABA. Unlike glutamate, it is inhibitory, and that in itself sheds light on how the brain works. Inhibition is the key to controlled action. By far most of the neurotransmitters latching onto a neuron's inputs tell it, "Don't fire." It's as though all the neurons in the brain had their firing hammers set, and just the right bursts to initiate a complex and precise action—a tiger springing, a composer humming—are brought about by blocking the circuits not wanted more than by tripping those needed to make it so. The analogy recalls Michelangelo's description of sculpting as cutting away stone to bring out forms within in the rock. GABA is the sculptor. But something happens to GABA or its receptor, Treiman says, that allows one circuit or all of them to fire without end. And the latter, the firing of all circuits, is the generalized status epilepticus Gail Beck suffered, the worst killer.

Treiman's published research asserts that generalized status epilepticus kills 50 percent of its victims unless they can be brought out of it quickly. Many survivors are vegetative, others left with little that could be called a meaningful quality of life.

Thinking of these ominous facts brings back a profoundly cautionary comment by Jeffrey Frank, the neurointensivist in charge of the University of Chicago NICU, on the power of modern medicine: "Sometimes we can enable our patients to survive with a disability beyond their worst nightmare."

EACH DAY AS MAYER led the team on rounds, there was Joe Beck, distraught but determined, with a thick notebook in hand and a dozen new questions. Ever more haggard, he took Mayer's answers down carefully. But the neurointensivist didn't have much to tell, other than to caution him that his wife's odds were looking worse. It was only after 14 days that he was able to bring Gail out of coma without her seizures recurring. But there was little sign of recovery. He had to let Joe know that there was a very real possibility Gail would glide into the death-in-life of the persistent vegetative state. Joe was in living hell.

From there Gail developed pneumonia and was pumped full of antibiotics, including antiviral acyclovir for the still-unconfirmed encephalitis. Her ventilator face mask was replaced with tracheostomy, a permanent air tube in her throat. IV feeding yielded to a PEG, a permanent feeding tube inserted through her stomach wall. *Permanent* is an ominous term in the ICU. Each of these decisions is a landmark one hopes not to reach.

Rashes indicated allergic reaction to one or more of her powerhouse drugs. Other drugs were mixed and matched to control it.

The seizures returned.

Mid-July: Seizures controlled for a time.

July 23: Up through the tight web of anticonvulsants burst new, "breakthrough seizures."

August 8: The NICU team had done all it could. Gail Beck was no longer in status; epilepsy is a chronic condition, and it was unclear what other aspects of her desperate condition were chronic. She was sent to Mount Sinai Rehabilitation Center.

August 8, same day: Back to Columbia Neuro ICU with uninterrupted seizing. On and on, up and down, lightning storms damping only to rekindle, without betraying a cause. This, Mayer told Joe, was the waiting game.

Joe was now looking back on summer with little more to recall than the NICU and the Long Island Expressway. Sixty-four round trips on the LIE, sometimes alone, sometimes with one or more of the family.

Jump to the end of the dramatic phase of the waiting game. Gail did not die, nor did she sink into a persistent vegetative state. On Wednesday, September 4, the first day of the new school year, Joe made the final trip to the NICU, to bring Gail "home," to the St. Charles Rehabilitation Center, two miles down the road in Melville. She had no muscle strength or energy so she could hardly walk, even with a walker. But she was going home. Her mother carried Ian in to reunite them. Gail looked up, burst into a grin. "What a beautiful baby!" she cried. "Whose is it?"

No memory. No bad memory of the summer, no good memory of the years behind, her long-term memory shot; perhaps she would have to begin again, laying down short term memories one by one. But there was something more, which many would consider the worst. She suffered from "flat affect," a common outcome of severe epilepsy when recognition does not bring along rich, layered feelings. Emotions are somehow tied into memory and perception in the region surrounding the hippocampus, and deep down in the hypothalamus, and perhaps deeper still in the adjoining thalamus, and it was not clear that she would ever regain them. Often she was in despair, and that represents feeling, but not necessarily feelings tagged onto the words and thoughts, faces, sounds that draw meaningful human life out of raw experience. She was alive and home again. Joe got his wish. Now what?

Possible outcomes of the waiting game: in addition to memory deficits there were language problems, called aphasias, of an astonishing variety, each a window into a part of the brain. Damage to Broca's area in the frontal lobe, in a region of the motor cortex across the valley from the temporal lobe, can leave the inability to speak, even though words are understood. Damage to a rear sector of the temporal lobe, called Wernicke's area and appropriately near the auditory cortex, can produce an inability to understand language. For most of us, these language areas are on the left side. But Johns Hopkins neurologist Argye Hillis points out that the right hemisphere, which we associate with global apprehending, gestalt, intuition rather than serial thinking, also has a language link. Those suffering right-brain damage often do not get the meaning of what is said. They may fail to understand emotional intonations, even though the sentences make perfect sense since their left brains are intact. For example, they may fail to get jokes. In a visual analog, they may not recognize emotion in facial expression. Hillis said one of her patients could perfectly describe a drawing on which she was tested. It showed a woman cooking at a stove, a nearby kitchen sink, a pot on the edge of the sink, and water flowing into and out of it. She could not apprehend the single thing the rest of us would spot at first glance: the pot is overflowing, flooding the kitchen floor. She got everything but the import.

IT IS FOUR SUMMERS LATER, 2000, when Stephan Mayer plops down the thick folder with Gail Beck's name on it and recounts her story. His colleague Stanley Resor has been Gail's epileptologist in all the years since, and Stephan only knows it's been some roller coaster for her. He hasn't seen her, has no idea how she is, how the Becks are doing. It's the nature of the job of the intensivist—the rescuer—to be left with little or no idea of the fate of patients unless they write or visit, and, since the patients usually remember little of their time in the NICU, that is rare. There was only a letter from Joe Beck in 1998 that began, "This is the saddest letter I have ever had to write. . . " and went on to detail the family's grinding financial straits and Gail's condition.

How could one measure her current condition? Mayer is particularly critical of the category-coded language of patient follow-ups that are written up in all branches of medicine. "The patient says, 'I feel fine, just like before, never better,' " Mayer says. "You talk to the wife alone and she says, 'He used to play with the kids, he worked like crazy, he loved sports. Now he just sits around the house all day watching whatever comes on TV.' But based on the guy's report, you could write him up as complete recovery. That's not what I call a good outcome."

Then he charges off to rounds again, into the thick of things. He is at the bedside of Michael Sanders, 45, the other half of the Long Island story. "Michael! Michael! Look at me! Show me two fingers! Look at me!" Mayer shouts to the impassive, clean-shaven face topped by curly, steel gray hair. Then to his team: "Not today I guess."

Rounding with Mayer are two medical students, three neurology residents, a new neurointensive fellow and—Mayer's godsend—the attending neurointensivist he just hired from Johns Hopkins who can spell him on call. Columbia's NICU has been run by a neurointensivist for as long as Johns Hopkins's, but there are key differences.

Columbia Neurology Chair Gerald Fink put the idea in place in 1983, but for many years he was sole attending and there was no training program. On the other hand, although in overall charge of the NICU, Fink did not manage neurosurgery patients, who usually account for the largest number in the unit. At Johns Hopkins, Dan Hanley did so. Because trained neurointensivists are so scarce, the Columbia "model" is by far the most common, but the Johns Hopkins program is often aspired to. Now Mayer has Ricardo Carhuapoma, fresh from Johns Hopkins, who will prove so smart and able as an attending that the chief of neurosurgery will be persuaded of the high value of neurointensivists, though no one would turn down any extra hands in the NICU.

Sanders remains unresponsive to each test of brain function. Lacking the blackened eyes or massive bandaging of the trauma or surgery patient, Sanders simply appears in a deep sleep from which he does not wake. But when Mayer presses a key into the bed of his thumbnail, Sanders's eyes slide half open, and he darts a quick glance toward the offending doctor. The movement, called a saccade, holds out hope there is not only a light on in there, but, deep down, someone *is* home. It is important that the saccade is in the direction of the pain, implying a brain stem that may be completely intact. As everyone knows firsthand, the whole of the "self" fades every night in sleep, when there may be only a dim sense of time passing, then it rises in an instant—or a bit longer for some—on waking. But anyone who has been knocked out by trauma or anesthesia knows that all consciousness vanishes completely, along with any sense of time passing. One moment is stitched directly to another that may be hours or days later in the "real world." But as long as the neurons are healthy and nourished and their circuits intact, life resumes without a glitch. That is, as long as the brain stem has been keeping the heart beating, blood circulating, lungs breathing and organs functioning.

Michael Sanders is here, breathing, by the slimmest of odds, and he is breathing only by virtue of the ventilator that also keeps his heart pumping blood to his brain and other vital organs. He faces no better odds of recovering, and Mayer has already braced his wife, Marybeth Collins, for the worst.

S HE IS DEVASTATED, Mayer says. "A guy in the prime of his life, married, two children. I had to discuss with her the real possibility that he will remain vegetative." Unknown to anyone, Sanders had an aneurysm on his middle cerebral artery. It hemorrhaged, and the shock to his brain caused his heart to stop. The hemorrhage now is contained, but death of brain tissue—infarction—remains a real possibility. He could be speechless in any combination of ways, because the middle cerebral artery nourishes the language areas, both for speaking and for understanding. He could be entirely disinhibited, losing every "social grace," if small parts of the forebrain are destroyed.

Michael Sanders, bank branch manager, was at home on a fine Father's Day, June 18, preparing to host a family barbeque. Late in the morning, he hopped in the car to run out for some last-minute refreshments and cigarettes, something a man with a time bomb in his brain definitely should not do. But he had no idea that the aneurysm was puffing out, like the ballooning of a weak inner tube.

At his neighborhood gas station Michael ordered his cigarettes from the attendant, who turned to pull them from the shelf and turned back to find the customer gone. Michael had collapsed. His heart had stopped cold, brought on by the aneurysm's leaking. Death would come in fewer minutes than an ambulance response, irreversible brain damage even quicker.

A few minutes earlier, Rose Estepa, a licensed practical nurse, and her 2-year-old daughter had been driving home from a Father's Day visit with Rose's father when they approached the gas station. She needed cigarettes before her shift at a retirement home and, as parents do, she thought out loud. "Wonder if I should stop now or wait?" Her daughter cried, "Mommy, stop now!" So for no better reason, Estepa did so, arriving at the cashier's window to find Michael Sanders lying on the ground.

Rushing to his side, she reached for his wrist. He had a pulse. Now he didn't, just like that. She immediately administered CPR, keeping his lungs inflated, and she had a pulse back when paramedics got there. About 80 percent of patients who go into cardiac arrest are DOA—dead on arrival—at the hospital. Sanders was among the lucky 20 percent. But now, more than three weeks later, he remained in a coma.

On the evening he had been brought to Columbia, Sanders had been taken into surgery to repair the aneurysm before it really blew and killed him on the spot. The cardiac arrest he'd suffered was a common one, Mayer knew, when an aneurysmal bleed hit neurons. A surge of excitatory catecholamine neurotransmitters was set loose, just as it would be if you turned a corner and saw a lion coming your way, and the immediate surge in blood pressure and demand on the heart was often too much. But Sanders was lucky in that regard. He may not have suffered any infarction of the heart muscle; once beating again, it might be good as new. His brain was something else again.

The most common way of preventing a bleeding aneurysm from rupturing is to place a very tiny clip over its neck, sealing the bulb off from the rest of the artery, just as you might seal the opening of a balloon with a clothespin. But in Sanders's case, instead of clipping, the neurosurgeon had sealed off the aneurysm with a coil. A fine metal wire was inserted through a catheter fed up through the femoral artery in the thigh. Once inside the aneurysm's bulb, the wire was fed out of the catheter and immediately twisted itself into loops, then tighter loops, and finally a glob of metal that stoppered the aneurysm at the neck. This required no opening of the skull.

What's the best method, to clip an aneurysm or coil it? That remains a major debate in the neuro world into the new century. Clipping an aneurysm, most neurosurgeons contend, is the most certain way of eliminating the potential for later complications; on the other hand, it requires arguably the most invasive surgery ever developed, beneath the skull and into the brain itself. By contrast, coiling requires no skull opening, so there are none of the risks of neurosurgery or deep anesthesia. But, "clippers" argue, many a coil has had to be replaced, repaired or retrieved because, over time, it stopped working.

Morning rounds are done, but Mayer never stops running. Up to the eighth floor, where his office sits tucked away in a narrow hall off the patient floor. He has business in both areas, in his office first.

Space is always at a premium in medical centers. The older the institution and the pricier its city's real estate, the tighter space becomes, which explains this tightest of warrens that is the administrative home to the Columbia NICU. Mayer's private office, tucked back to the right from the front door, is just big enough for him and one visitor. Tucked to the left of Mayer's office is Carhuapoma's. And behind the administrative assistant at the door, on the far side of a head-high divider, is an area almost entirely consumed by a long conference table and chairs. But there are still more small desks and chairs scattered for research directors, assistants.

While he waits for the brother of a very sick patient out on the eighth floor to come by, Mayer pulls out materials for the most important organizational work he's up to right now: forming the Neurocritical Care Society. This group—still a shell, a concept—represents the aspirations of most of the trained neurointensivists in the country. Ultimately they would like board certification as the third subspecialty of neurology, to take their place in full view of the important medical associations, insurance payers and hospital administrations. They would join pediatric neurologists and neurophysiologists, the epilepsy specialists.

None of this seems important for most of us, not worth a candle of attention compared with the dramatic duties of a neurointensivist. But to medical administrators like Mayer and Mirski, such recognition can mean the difference between progress for their subspecialty and its fading away—which, to them, would mean a great deal to patient care. But no one argues this: long-term goals take a backseat to the urgent, as chronic problems wait behind the acute. And the most dramatic of urgent problems came to Mayer right now, as a page from the floor. Antonia Gonzalez's brother has arrived.

Antonia has made her wishes known to her family, and those wishes have been passed on to Mayer by her brother. She is a lifelong paraplegic and has been quadriplegic for the last few years. If anything happened that would bring her even lower—dim her consciousness, remove the spark of love and communication with her family—she wanted to be taken off life support. That time has come. Mayer would do so.

Intubation and extubation—inserting and removing the ventilator tube from a patient's airway—are learned skills. Taking a patient off life-support—terminal extubation—adds a profoundly troubling dimension to the act. How does a physician prepare for such decisions as terminal extubation, let alone teach others to make them? The answer is a bit chilling. "Our patients are our teachers," Mayer says. "We are doing things so cutting-edge, neither we nor anybody else has reams of experience. So we try to make the best, smartest decisions we can, by consensus. Keep talking till we all agree." But he admits that "sometimes you just don't get everybody on the same page." Importantly, the family has made this decision with unanimity, and, unusually, Antonia had made her wishes clear long ago. Mayer was meeting with her brother to tell him it was time. Opposition to terminal extubation. Mayer says, comes most often from other physicians, who believe it is a violation of their Hippocratic oath to take such an active role in ending a human life.

Now it is time for afternoon rounds in the NICU, and they have hardly begun when a faraway monitor goes into a bizarre musical cadence that makes it stand out from all the others. To calm the ICU, monitor alarms have been toned down from the old wailing sirens and clanging bells. The results, if not jarring, are no less attention-getting. This one sounds like a kazoo whose mad player sings obsessively into it, Hum-ho, hum-ho. But now plays it louder. Ever louder and with more feeling: HO-hum HO-HO-HO, HO-hum HO-HO-HO, HO-hum HO-HO-HO.

And on that cue a nurse hurries up and says in an easy, steady voice, "There's an emergency in Room 4, please."

The kazoo's manic singsong grows louder as Mayer leads the team into Michael Sanders's room. He and resident Stacy Wu quickly pull bright yellow infection gowns just over their forearms and yank on rubber gloves.

"Something is clogging his lungs," Mayer says as the nurse suctions the tube already inserted in his throat. Michael twists and stretches on the bed, head of steel gray hair moving side to side. He is strangling. As his lungs are cleared, he quiets. So does the kazoo. *Hum-ho, hum-ho.*

Mayer reviews charts and drugs with Wu, since she is the resident following this case. She rattles off Sanders's vital signs and prescriptions. Mayer makes changes, then says, looking at her, "Would someone stay with him please? Let's go."

In moments like these, the neurointensivist's most common theme, that the need for hands-on action led them here, seems inarguable. But what about other neurologists? Where are the pipe smokers? Fisher's endowed chair at Stanford Medical Center provides him funds and time for research to keep on the cutting edge of neurophysiology. But he also sees patients, on many days from morning until night, in clinic, or, for those in status epilepticus, in the Neuro ICU. He is so busy, all the time, that his cool makes it clear that he has his hurricane of a schedule in perfect control. He has just become the editor of *Epilepsia,* considered one of two top journals in this specialty. This, he points out, will put him in the center of things, make him better able to keep up on the latest big ideas—including, he hopes, the off-center ideas that a more senior editor might too quickly dismiss. He may be able to influence, to guide, as well as to discover—taken together, perhaps an academic physician's defining ambition.

So where is the distanced, cerebral, aloof neurologist? Granted that the in-house jokes among doctors are no less stereotyped than others', you will not meet a 9-to-5-er among the many neurologists enountered in this story. Is there a genuine distinction to be made here between these

neurologists and the intensivists? Or has that urge to pigeonhole hard-
ened a blurry difference, created a false distinction?

Not according to Timothy Pedley, Columbia's chair of neurology, "and
I'm not only a neurologist, I'm an epileptologist," he says. And an
M.D./Ph.D. to boot, who was a benchmate of Fisher's during their doctoral
work—crossing pathways again.

Other neurologists may work hard, he says, but there is a critical leap
in "this new generation of neurologist" as intensivist.

"They've moved from hands-off, consultative work that neurologists
traditionally do to hands-on, interventional decisionmaking," Pedley says.
"That's a huge difference, and the personal cost to those who do it is very
high." Noting that the founders of the subspecialty are no longer practicing in it, he says, "You leave that field in midcareer. The emotional stress
levels are too high." Columbia's Fink now is president of Mount Sinai
Medical Center. Hanley has gone full bore into research on brain injury
outcomes. Allan Ropper, who created the course that gave birth to the
field at Massachusetts General Hospital, is chief of neurology at St.
Elizabeth's Medical Center, a teaching hospital in Boston. Ropper says of
the specialization he spearheaded, for which he wrote the first textbook:
"It's a young man's game."

The compelling, driving force in the intensivists' day, as they tell it
themselves, is rescue. Every patient in the unit is in danger of dying, some
more so, some less, but otherwise they wouldn't be here. The compelling,
driving force in *all* academic neurology is research: finding answers that
will eliminate the need for rescue, or that will assure rescue, or that will
restore the human beings rescued to the ones who set out on the odyssey
where we enounter them. There is one goal on every odyssey, the same as
on the first such voyage that gave all the rest its name: to get home again,
restored to the condition in which you left. But for their doctors, only the

Iliad offers even a limited model. Each of them is making a war that only carries forward, each with different goals and some with opposing visions.

However, all the doctors in this story are also academics, and that unites them perhaps as much as their specialties. The academy prescribes a major presence in the laboratory as well as in the clinic. And this is no secret: first, research; second, clinic. That is how medical faculty are judged from Harvard, Johns Hopkins, Columbia, and Stanford to every leading academic medical center. The neurointensivist lives most truly in the clinic, the NICU, so he or she often is more conflicted than counterparts in many other neuro subspecialties when facing the demands of research. The proximity of Michael Sanders in this bed and of Antonia, his NICU neighbor just yesterday, raises this question: If Michael were to die, how would we know? It is a question every NICU physician must not merely ask, but decide. In the age of the ventilator, death does not come because it is observed, but because it is decided. David Beyda, a medical ethicist at Georgetown University and the head of a pediatrics intensive care unit himself, puts this the most dramatically: "If you are a patient in my ICU, you cannot die unless I say you can die. And then you will die when I say, on my schedule." It is not an opinion or a decision of Beyda's that this be so. It is a fact of life he will not let anyone forget.

So the answer is that, because of this great technology, Michael Sanders cannot die unless Mayer lets him. But that doesn't mean he can really live, that his life will have meaning for him or anyone else.

Michael will get better, wife Marybeth says with simple conviction. She is an executive with a corporation that owns hotels throughout the United States and not someone given to superstition, but she does believe that sometimes there are signs. She pulls a picture from a photo package. The day after Michael's attack, these pictures came back from the lab, she says. They were taken at a local veterans' hall.

The picture shows Sanders leaning over a pool table, cue poised, smiling out at Marybeth, at us. Behind him, caught by chance, is the bottom of a veterans' memorial banner hanging on the wall. The words encircle Michael's head like a medieval halo:

You are not forgotten.

For Marybeth, this is sign enough.

Stephan Mayer wants other signs but does not find them. Yet in his own way he is as much a believer, an optimist.

Maybe it's a hunch, he says at the end of the day, but I think Michael is going to walk out of here. Wake up and walk out. He is speaking to new colleagues around a little table in the Turning Leaf Café as afternoon draws to a close. A sweet, pastoral image that, but the Turning Leaf is a collection of tables scattered across the polished stone of the multistory entrance foyer of New York Presbyterian Hospital, looking out toward Fort Washington Avenue. Like every coffee break for the neurointensivist, this one marks a loosening of the intellectual grip just to get a different hold on things. He is briefing them on their role in the Neuro ICU.

At any given time Johns Hopkins has six or seven neurointensivists rotating as attending physicians in managing the Neuro ICU, plus four fellows—two senior, two junior—and various residents from neurology and neurosurgery on critical care rotations. Until last week, Columbia had one attending physician, Mayer, and no fellow. Even though he does not manage every patient in the unit, he is on constant first call, nights and weekends.

"There is no case in this unit where I can say, Not mine," Mayer says to his colleagues, a critical point because many ICUs are territorial, with each specialist commanding care for his or her patients. Ricardo

Carhuapoma, having just arrived from Johns Hopkins to be co-attending, already knows this as gospel.

Mayer: "You need to feel a sense of responsibility for everyone. And that means 16 very sick patients. For a given bedside procedure, I may do it, the neurosurgery resident may do it, but I'm responsible. You need a global sense of responsibility."

Into the early summer evening of a long day, Mayer explains to his new team members how to traverse the difficult terrain of admitting patients while on duty alone at night. What do you say if the patient has no insurance? What do you say if there are insurance questions you cannot answer? If it's a transfer from another hospital, another state? If there's no room? If room could be made? A tortuous conversation peppered with "But you'll get used to it," and "It's not so hard."

It sure sounds hard, negotiating and bargaining in the middle of the hard night.

He urges those taking call to phone him at any hour if need be but, in the ironic manner of the intense, he says of himself and his rheumatologist wife, Elizabeth, "We have a four-month-old baby sleeping in bed with us, so midnight calls are sub-optimal. If I wake the baby, I may be invited to the couch."

But these days Mayer, the head of this major unit at the age of 37, is a young physician with a new spring in his step, a lightened load. Until a few days ago, in an emergency in the middle of any night, there was no one else *to* call. Mayer was the lone attending neurointensivist for the entire unit. Now there are two, and a fellow in the bargain.

IT'S ALWAYS RUSH HOUR on the Long Island Expressway, and the feeder highway off of it is also heavy with traffic, leading right to the door of the Becks' duplex across the street from a pocket shopping center.

Gail answers the door, apologizes for the tumble of boxes and housewares, toys scattered in the living room. They are moving in two weeks. She is, on first meeting, a "regular person." There is nothing in her speech or manner that suggests she has survived a devastating illness. Joe gives a hearty greeting and handshake, and it's clear from his tone, his words, that he feels they are delivered. Gail is less sure, quick to be annoyed with herself. "I used to love *Hamlet*," she says. "I can't concentrate anymore. I'm trying to get through *The Godfather* now, and that's tough enough."

"It's a start!" Joe counters, encouragingly.

The boys shyly say hello. Gail says they've been terrific about her recurrent seizures. "I'll be sitting on the couch and slump over, and they know to call my sister and not to worry," she says. "The seizures aren't bad. I usually just fade out, like falling asleep for a few minutes. Every now and then I have a worse one and wake up on the floor. Usually, I can get to the couch. But I guess what gets to me most is my memory. Sometimes it seems I can't remember anything."

Her frustrations seem small by comparison with what her prospects had been, but they are sharp all the same. "I know this will sound crazy to most women, but I just wish I could do my own shopping. I would love to drive again. I could drive the boys around; I could shop by myself."

At this, or at any hint of pessimism, Joe looks heavenward, shakes his head. Deliverance. He is teaching English at nearby Plainview High School. He has written a play, and in its depiction of an elderly husband's efforts to cope with his wife's Alzheimer's, it's clear he is exorcising the early years of recovery when Gail's memory really was shot, when everything looked dark. They've been seeing epileptologist Stanley Resor at Columbia for four years now. First this medication, now that one; a new combination. Two years ago they went to the Mayo Clinic in Rochester, Minnesota, as long a trip as Gail has ever taken. Ups, downs. She tries not to get discouraged. "I try to take it a little bit at a time," she says. True, as you listen to her, there is a slow, measured texture to her speech that suggests someone on tranquilizers. But someone all there, for sure.

IN HIS COLUMBIA OFFICE, Resor flips the pages of Gail's life, as measured in dosages of medications with arcane, tongue-twisting names. Gail's seizures, he is sure, had a multifocal onset, then became generalized and progressed to status epilepticus. Reflecting on the fact that she cried out as she first seized, he says it is common for a seizure to strike the motor cortex region controlling the diaphragm or the throat's glottis, yielding an involuntary cry or loud moan. She has auras, premonitions of a seizure coming, also a sign of focal rather than generalized seizure at the start. "Primary generalized seizures are usually genetic" in origin, he says. Still, Gail's auras are not well focused. Some patients have auras so clear, with such precise timing, that they can drive, knowing they will be prompted by the clockwork aura minutes before a seizure to pull off the road.

Tall and lanky, Resor slouches in his chair, seven o'clock on a Friday night and the last patient just gone. "Phenobarbital at first, but that's a barbiturate, so it's addictive," he says as he reads from Gail's file. "If you withdraw it suddenly, you can give a seizure to someone who's never had one." He carefully picks his way through the field of possibilities, many discovered serendipitously. "Valproic acid is a solvent. In the early sixties it was used to dissolve seizure-inducing drugs being given to test animals. None of them had seizures. Someone figured out it was the solvent." That's now called Depakote, one of the major antiseizure drugs. He doesn't like Depakote compared with others, not long term, so he works to get his patients off it if he can. Balancing this panoply of drugs and doses underscores what skills are

needed to be an epileptologist, other than correctly interpreting a seemingly impenetrable EEG printout.

"Phenobarbital makes the body get rid of Depakote quickly," he says.
"So you have to give a bigger dose of Depakote if it's in combination." A
pause. "But Depakote makes it *harder* for the body to get rid of phenobarbital, so if you're not careful you wind up with too big a dose of phenobarbital."

A bit of this, a jolt of that. This is the high-art end of the medical spectrum, empirical to the core. True, a new drug protocol may emerge from
clinical trials as "evidence-based medicine," but it takes far more than for-
mulas and error bars to make it all work. Resor points out that only two
seizure medications were developed from scratch—that is, with their
mechanisms of action known from the start. The others were developed
for other purposes, such as sedation. Their effects suggested a benefit in
seizure control, and trials confirmed it.

Even so, the preferences of epileptologists vary more radically than,
say, favoring mannitol over salt solution in the NICU. Resor dislikes one
of the hot new drugs on the market because "it makes people stupid." On
the other hand, he likes Lamictal, which "scared off lots of U.S. doctors"
after it was introduced from Great Britain. It gave some patients severe
rashes of the epithelium, the lining of the mouth and throat, of blood vessels, and of such inner organs as the liver and kidneys. The kidney rashes
proved fatal in some cases. But Resor says such side effects can be completely prevented. "You start slower, monitor very closely, and look for
signs of oral rash." Gail has been doing well on Lamictal, which has fewer
side effects than many other drugs.

Phenobarbital reduces the effectiveness of Lamictal, so once Resor
was able to get Gail off phenobarbital, the Lamictal's effectiveness in-

creased. "But when I stop the Depakote, that will make Lamictal levels drop, so I'll have to increase it." And on through the maze.

A YEAR HAS GONE BY since the Becks loaded up all those boxes and moved a few miles away to their new home, in a quiet neighborhood of Bethpage. Long gone is *The Godfather*, but Gail is not yet ready for *Hamlet*. Gone, too, is the flat, emotionless voice that had marked her as she left Columbia and whose traces remained even a year ago. She laughs a lot. Her sense of humor is keen. She plays on words.

She still has seizures. "Not as bad as before," she says. "And the boys are great about it." Her big leap forward: she must still be driven to the store, but she can take care of all the shopping herself, preparing the list, remembering where to find everything. She loves the new house, really loves the neighborhood. Her next goal is to stencil borders atop the dining room walls. Her mother doesn't want her to do it alone, afraid she will fall off the ladder, but Gail is certain enough of her auras not to be worried. Lately, she has never failed to make it to the couch when she felt a seizure coming on.

"Part of my frustration is that I'm very competitive," she says. "I can't stand to lose." But now she is losing at chess, not the simple board games of a year ago. At first, playing with 11-year-old Andrew—who is, she admits, a very good chess player and as competitive as she is—Gail was losing consistently. Now she beats him often enough. A big roll of the eyes from Joe.

Sometimes she feels those auras, a sense of fading, while she is playing chess and thinking about the many possible moves ahead, hopping in her mind among alternatives. Sometimes it's in big family gatherings, like Thanksgiving, when many people are talking in cross-conversation and she is trying to thread her way among them. "I just pull back a while. I'll go take it easy, by myself, for a few minutes, and it goes away."

Her memory may skip a few beats now and then, but never her will and self-direction. Here she is walking Ian to the school bus for his first day of kindergarten. One minute, there they are. The next, she's looking at the sky as the gurney is being loaded into an ambulance. "I'm telling them, 'Stop, I'm okay. Just leave me, I'm fine.' But, no, they had to take me." She is determined that, with her prodding, anyone who knows her will, like Andrew and Ian, not worry if she fades out for a few moments.

Time heals. Medicine heals. Neither works all the time. Which is the tonic for Gail Beck? Hard to tell, say Mayer and Resor. Only the outcome is clear. A few weeks after Mayer had brought out her thick, years' old file in his office, Gail and Joe walked into the NICU for the first time since she had gone home. Nurses flocked toward her, weeping with joy. Gail, who was meeting them for the first time, couldn't help but join in.

"IF YOU MET ME when I was at Columbia, then you know I don't remember you," he says sardonically. "In fact, I don't remember Columbia. It's as if I was never there."

Michael Sanders and wife Marybeth Collinis are having brunch at a diner near their home in Massapequa, on the South Shore. He is wearing a Jets football jacket, jeans, athletic shoes, but Marybeth is dressed for business, will leave here for work. At the start, Michael seems in the grip of the restless anger that strikes the laid-off or newly retired. Inactivity is getting to him. "I'm anxious to get back to work," he says, "And I will get back to work. I've been a banker my whole adult life and I don't intend to quit now." But in Marybeth's eyes shows not sympathy or agreement, or even exasperation, but real anxiety. Soon it becomes clearer. Michael is angry at everything.

The Jets have just fired the coach. "That was stupid, but then everything they do is stupid." Not said with the crooked smile of a fan. Yet *not really pissed off.* His voice remains flat. The words are angry, the voice is nondescript. In some ways reminiscent of Dana Carvey's "angry old man," Michael is angry, in a way, at everything you can name. Angry with the bank that will not take him back, *but they better.* Angry that he cannot concentrate, cannot do math with the fluid skill he always could, and him a banker. Angry at being stuck at home. Angry at—Go ahead, name something. Yet unlike Gail Beck, he is never searching for a word or a name. His speech is as fluent as it must always have been. Place names, directions, everything rapid-fire.

Marybeth says nothing until later, on the phone. "He plans things but can't do them. He understands exactly what he needs to do most of the time, but he can't motivate himself to follow through. So he sits in the house all day."

Mixing memory and desire . . . What Michael needs to do is to take logical, orderly steps, well-learned and clearly remembered by the "cold" rational brain, in order to take himself into a desired future. Nothing seems damaged in the recall or the reasoning. What has been lost appears to be at the level of emotion and feeling, the realm of one of the most primitive parts of our brain, the limbic system. *Desire.* That makes all the difference, as though each tiny element of rational thought needed to be powered on its pathway to choice, toward action, by a hunger for an end.

Does the powering of "rational thinking" by "gut feelings" somehow become what we call the will? Something like that emerges from recent work by Antonio Damasio and others, studying brain-injured patients whose reasoning appears intact but whose motivation is severely diminished or absent. Damasio is head of Neurology at the University of Iowa, a prominent neuroscientist and a best-selling author on the subject. In *Descartes' Error,*

Damasio argued that the great philosopher had committed a fundamental error by dividing the human mind into twin entities—the animal soul that provides feeling and emotion, rage, brute love; and the rational soul that guides and drives human achievement. In case after case of his own patients, Damasio offers powerful evidence that the truth is closer to the opposite, that it is the "feel" of what is right that leads us to choose, in thousands of decisions big and small that make up a typical day of choices and actions.

Time heals, medicine heals, just not all ways. A year later, Michael and Marybeth are in the final stages of divorce. It would have been over long ago, he says in his apartment in Massapequa, if she weren't playing so many games, she and her lawyer. He is angry, but that's certainly common enough in divorce. He is perfectly rational in explaining. Is he angrier than most? If the words he speaks this winter afternoon were written down, quote by quote, you might think he was someone prone to violence. But to think that, you would have to invest his words with passion. Such variations in emotional coloring have bred utterly different Hamlets out of the same written words, over four centuries with no end in sight. Sanders's voice is no longer flat, but its coloration is conversational. You can hear the same tones over the same issues from a cab driver, a bar patron. There is no body language, not a wave of the arm, not a flip-off finger at the world, at lawyers—nothing, but maybe that's always been him.

The apartment is neat, sparsely furnished. There are numerous golf trophies in one room. He has always been a good golfer, he says, regularly beating his friends. Now they won't play with him anymore. "I've gotten better since my accident," he says. "I think my swing is more relaxed."

Told this is a nice place, he sneers. He hates it, hates Massapequa. He cannot stand the South Shore. People on the South Shore are uniformly ignorant. He is from the North Shore, born in Huntington Hospital, stuck here for the time being.

Sanders is certainly rational: His sister, a nurse, told him that given his attack and his medications, alcohol would kill him. He has not had a drink in more than a year since. He says he had been an alcoholic since his teenage years. No more. He is glad to be divorcing, hated marriage. Why did he get married? "I was thirty. I figured, 'I'm thirty, it's time to get married.'" Nothing more? "Nothing."

Was there nothing more? Or is there only now nothing more, a memory stripped of its feeling? Who could know? One might describe desire as thought of a future moment soaked in "feeling good," a lure. If Michael feels such desire, nothing shows.

Marybeth has custody of the children. He threatened to kill her, over and over. He would say how much pleasure it would give him to kill her. That was when he was drinking so heavily, after he got home from the hospital. Damage to the amygdala, another part of that emotion-driving limbic system, can trigger outbursts of rage, especially in men, but it isn't clear there's any connection here. Marybeth finally got an order of protection against Michael, but had it lifted so he could come over and take the children for visits. Over lunch, near her Manhattan office, she reflects. Was he an alcoholic? She doesn't think so, not before the accident. But he did drink too much, in that she agrees with him. Was he so angry? Threatening? No. He had a temper. Maybe things were never quite right, maybe he always expected too much. But he was never like this.

Michael not only sounds like he's normal—if angry—he has in significant ways proved it. His bank's insurance company neurologist gave him the usual battery of tests, and he passed with flying colors. "So now he's off disability, living on unemployment," Marybeth says. That will run out in a few months. She has told him he should fight the disability ruling, that he is not ready to work, and Michael says he will, but he does not. She points out that he not only speaks at a very high level but reads well, though she is not certain he remembers what he has read, or that he is able to "juggle the facts" that he reads or remembers.

Within months he has moved again, to nearby Lindenhurst, but now is preparing to move yet again because he doesn't like his landlord.

"I wish things hadn't turned out like this, but I wish him well, I really do, " she says later on the phone. "I hope he figures out what he wants."

REFLECTING ON SANDERS'S state of mind, Stephan Mayer offers some provocative observations of his former patient, whom he has not seen in years. Michael Sanders's injury came two years after Gail Beck's, almost to the day. Maybe, despite what appears to be such a critical, permanent loss, Michael is just like Gail Beck at the same stage of recovery. That period would be 1998, when Joe Beck wrote "the saddest letter I have ever had to write."

Months later, Michael is answering questions again, on the phone. He still has not appealed his disability denial, though he intends to. His old list of complaints seems no shorter. But he is assistant coach for his son's Little League team. He rattles off with impressive ease the ways he has instructed the boy to play first base in a variety of scenarios. There does, indeed, seem to be feeling in his voice, perhaps a sense of humor. Who knows but Michael? It's easy to invest these qualities where they aren't and to miss them when they're plain as day.

CHAPTER 6

A Model Universe

"A failed experiment is not one that shows a
treatment to be of no value. A failed experiment
is one that does not give a clear answer."
—ROBERT S. FISHER, M.D./PH.D.
July 2001

LONG WHITE RAT lies on its side in the mini OR, its nose stretched into a clear plastic cylinder that delivers a precise dosage of halothane or isofluorane, the same anesthetics used in Johns Hopkins Hospital across the street, from tanks at the foot of the operating table. A few feet above the still form, heating lamps glow red, bright against the summer morning light that reflects through the large, dusty window facing north from the Traylor research building. Dr. Tommy Toung, gowned, masked and gloved, makes a slit incision in the rat's scalp, then drills a small burr hole in its skull. Anish Bhardwaj stands at his side, holding the microdialysis tube Toung will insert, and outlines the experiment.

Inside the plastic tube is a catheter about the thickness of a human hair, and it will be slipped under the rat's brain-enveloping meninges. Then Toung will stitch the flap closed to prevent infection. The opposite end of the fine catheter feeds into a test tube. Slender as the catheter is, however, inside it nests an entire experimental apparatus. First, there is a mesh bucket of netting so fine it will allow passage of only very tiny particles—molecules of neurotransmitters and their breakdown products, but not of the large chains of proteins. A human hair is about 750 microns thick; the whole bucket is less than half that. The bucket in turn is lidded, and through the lid are pressed two tubes so much finer still that they run side by side, with room to spare between them.

The experimenters now pump artificial cerebrospinal fluid down one of the tubes. It floods into the rat's brain, forcing out the animal's own CSF, which passes through the mesh and up the outflow tube. Those particles small enough to pass through the membranous net will be collected with the fluid in the test tube. They represent baseline data on the excitatory and inhibitory neurotransmitters circulating in this one rat's brain at an ordinary moment under anesthesia.

Later today, Toung will induce a stroke in the rat by blocking one of the key arteries in a blood vessel structure called the circle of Willis, a structure that we share, with variations, with all other mammals. Then he will carefully repeat the neurotransmitter collection to learn more about the effects of excitotoxicity on the brain of a mammal at precise intervals after a stroke occurs. The results of many such experiments on many such animals may clarify the pathway of ischemic destruction in ways that will lead from here across the street, to human stroke victims. That, at least, is the point of the experiment, and something like it is at the heart of all animal experimentation in medical research. Toung and Bhardwaj are at work in the laboratory of David Sherman, Ph.D., a biomedical engineer whose career is focused on the electrochemistry of the brain and the reading of its signals. He is their lab host and research partner.

A S T H E Y W O R K , Marek Mirski leaves his office to join them, navigating a typically labrinthine hospital path of a quarter mile. From Meyer 8, he traverses six large buildings, drops five flights and climbs three, and crosses one bridge—offering a gunsight view of the distant Washington Monument between Hopkins's towers—before swinging into the suite of labs that includes Dave Sherman's. He greets everyone and heads to the desk where Sherman leafs through a lab notebook.

Mirski is out of the NICU this week. That doesn't trim his administrative duties, which are much on his mind this month, but it does offer him a chance to get into the laboratory. The experiment Mirski and Sherman are running occupies another long table loaded with gear. Sherman, of medium height with a salt-and-pepper crew cut, is the principal investigator on an NIH grant that not only keeps his lab in business but funds Mirski's research within it. A major goal for Mirski is to secure an independent NIH award that will allow him, Sherman and Wendy Ziai to pursue this work and to contribute to the support of Sherman's lab. That notwithstanding, Mirski proudly points to his unit as bringing in as much NIH funding as any comparable group in the country, well ahead of the average for neurologists. Ziai comes in soon after and begins prepping test tubes on the far side of the room for the day's work.

In the center of the table where Mirski and Sherman lean is the dramatic focus of their attention. Another white rat darts or runs flat out within a two foot, clear plastic bowl. But the rat does not move with respect to us, the bowl does—spinning, stopping, and reversing according to the rat's motions. The bowl is on a turntable, a horizontal version of the "rat race" cage. The reason for the elaborate construction is to hold steady the tube that runs from a mini–gantry crane overhead straight down into the animal's skull. The tube contains the same device Bhardwaj and Toung are implanting, a microdialysis catheter, whose mesh similarly will allow passage of neurotransmitters and their by-products at varying intervals. A video camera is perched at an angle nearby, with an associated monitor and tape deck plugged into the assembly. Over by the window, Bhardwaj and Toung work on a model of stroke; here, Mirski, Ziai and Sherman on a model of seizure. The video demonstrating the animal's visible states of generalized seizure will be time-linked to the recording of neurotransmitters thrown off in its brain. Tied up right here is nearly 20 years of Mirski's life as the scientist half of his profession of clinician-investigator. Tied up, too, is a promising tool developed as a result of his investigations that is now in clinical trials, and thereby hangs a tale of doing science, long term. Mirski began his career in a lab much like this one, carrying out the experiments that were forerunners of those they are working on today.

WHEN MAREK MIRSKI ARRIVED at Johns Hopkins to begin residency in 1987, he brought with him a tantalizing series of findings that had earned his newly minted Ph.D. at Washington University. Tantalizing because they hinted at answers to some of the deepest questions in the neuroscience of epilepsy: Where are the origins of seizures that *start* as generalized, storming throughout the entire double hemisphere of the human cortex at once? That is, what deep brain structures are involved at the eruption of generalized seizures? What are the seizures' mechanisms of reinforcement and, more important, of control?

Generalized seizures are the most dangerous because they are global, although they are usually self-limiting and relatively few go on to become status epilepticus. *Self-limiting* means that controls must come into play. Such global seizures come in two forms, as we've seen. Sometimes they begin in one focus—often in the temporal lobe—and then spread throughout the brain, crossing the fibers of the corpus callosum that link the two hemispheres. These are the "secondarily generalized." But some seizures begin their rhythmic storms all over the brain at once. It was these "primary generalized" seizures that interested Mirski.

How is such a simultaneous eruption possible? Picturing a circuit amplified out of control and entraining others offers a simple metaphor for a focal seizure spreading to generalized. But the key to primary generalized seizures is that the thick carpet of neurons plunges communicating roots down to the center of the brain, and similar fibers rise upward from the central brain stem, radiating through that whole cortical surface. The sites for the electrical eruptions that could set off everything atop at once, therefore, must lie somewhere beneath the lobes of the forebrain—but where? Well before the middle of the twentieth century, many researchers thought the candidate best fitting the evidence was the thalamus, the twinned, egg-shaped cluster of deep-brain neurons that sits right at the juncture of the primitive brain stem and the large forebrain.

The thalamus fascinated Mirski. "Basically, you have a whole complex set of signals coming upward from the brain stem, the oldest part of the brain that is very little changed from the brains of very primitive animals. And you have a whole different set of signals coming down from the neocortex, the modern brain—a lot of it uniquely human brain. They operate in a kind of push-pull, and in many ways counter to one another." Much of the time, the commands learned by the cortex serve to override the signals from the brain stem, he says. If we're hit and tumble, for example, the brain stem signals us to thrust our hands out. Young football players are taught to override that and aim their helmets into a groundward skid, clutching their hands to midsection with the football tucked in, a very noninstinctive response. Pinch patients under a light anesthetic and they will, slumberously, lift a hand and push away the offending touch. Do the same to those whose brain stems alone remain active and they will stick one or both hands straight out—called extending.

Those two worlds, ancient mammal and modern human, meet right in the thalamus, where the single structures of the brain stem emerge into the dual hemispheres of the upper brain. It is the thalamus that must mediate the interchange of signals down—thoughts, sentiments, willing, wanting—to the viscera and limbs. And it is the thalamus that mediates the primitive apprehension of, say, life-threatening danger up into the thinking brain. Joined to it, the hypothalamus relays and modulates anger, joy, sex drive, and others of the most powerful integrated emotion-response complexes in the human personality, and it is the communicator with the body's master gland, the pituitary, which dangles beneath on its stalk.

Integration of various senses and emotions, in fact, seems the best short summary of what goes on within these two structures that collectively are called the diencephalon. One example hints at the power within this crossroads metropolis. The visual data set relayed from the retinas toward the rear-most occipital lobes in many ways mirrors the seen world: the lenses focus incoming "pictures" point for point against the retinas, and point for point the retinas send all the signals rearward. How does the brain reintroduce the original topography, the shape and relationship of each bit, for processing by the cortex? Much of that occurs where the optic nerves dive into the thalamus, emerging to join the occipital lobes on the final path toward making sense of it all.

The thalamus was a good suspect for the origin of generalized seizures, if indeed there was only one, but no one had proved it was ever such a seizure source. So, in 1982, Mirski set out, for his Ph.D. dissertation, to study the pathways of generalized seizures that could be induced chemically. The lab in which he carried out this work was under the direction of James Ferrendelli. Mirski constructed a model that he hoped would tell a truth that could be generalized from the brains of lower mammals to our own.

But before getting to his experiments, maybe we should ask a fundamental question. Why would anyone believe that learning a truth about an animal's brain would offer any valid information about our own?

Eric Kandel, who won a Nobel Prize for his work elucidating the pathways of learning in all brains by studying those in a primitive sea slug, offers the most general answer in *Principles of Neural Science*. "In the mid–nineteenth century, Charles Darwin set the stage for the study of animals as models of human actions and behavior by publishing his observations on the continuity of species in evolution." That continuity eventually gave rise to "the study of human and animal behavior under controlled conditions." The last phrase is the key to the unique structure that underlies nearly all modern science, a gift of such Renaissance "architects" as Galileo: the laboratory. And the controls painstakingly developed in the laboratory over centuries are the key to the extension of the lab experiment that underlies nearly all medical science: the clinical trial. *Careful observations by a prepared investigator carried out under controlled conditions* wraps into one expression three phrases heard throughout the world of science. The underlying assumption is that the motley world "out there" can, with enough care, be abstracted "in here," and in here studied, quantified, measured, made better food for thought.

Four centuries after Galileo and one and a half after Darwin, with the sun of Baltimore washing a patina of window shapes over cages and jars and the apothecary of a neuro lab, very little has changed at the core. Scientists want proof, but the bottom line is, they never get it. They know they will never get it. We all learn that science deals with uncertainties. Scientists get evidence, which comes from quantifying, often the previously unquantifiable, and then measuring what they have quanitifed. They hope their conclusions eventually will be persuasive, then convincing, maybe even overwhelming. The yield is truths that are real and important, that bring the world into ever clearer, sharper focus and allow diseases to be cured or averted. But these truths never integrate into smooth, uppercase Truth. They accrete more like wind arrows on a weather chart that, when all goes well, show pretty much the same direction. Just how precisely "pretty much" can be interpreted is also quantified, as various categories of error. No experimental measurement is more important than error. And the idea that quantifying error is *of the essence* owes to that earliest era of science, although the means for doing so have become a whole lot more sophisticated and the results more complex, harder to read.

W H I C H   B R I N G S   U S   B A C K   to Mirski's doctoral research: just because there is a continuum of "brain" from rodent to human does not mean that what is true of one's brain holds for the other's. The limitations and vagaries of animal model results are legion, and that fact helps to explain the path, far more tortuous than the walk from the NICU to this lab, that Mirski's work would take from its beginnings to the here and now. But it is important to notice that it is the researcher in the clinician-investigator most frustrated by limitations on animal models of human epilepsy. The physician celebrates if animal trials lead to improved patient care, even if the results are not crystal clear.

Mirski still has an album that, like a travelogue, displays the sequential films of his journey through the maze of the rodent brain that led him deep into its thalamus. His voyage is traced on X ray film rather than Kodachrome, and what glows out at us are the bright lights of radioactive molecules that settled in the animals' brains and eventually told him part of the story. *Eventually* and *part* are key.

Experiments with chemicals known to induce generalized seizures in animals had pointed to the involvement of deep brain structures, including the thalamus. How these chemicals work in itself indicates the nature of epilepsy's potential causes. The antibiotic penicillin applied directly to an animal's cortex will induce seizures, apparently by affecting the neuronal membrane and working against the inhibitory neurotransmitter GABA. That was also the effect of the chemical metrazol that Mirski used as convulsant in his experiments.

He wanted to know what pathways were "lit up," or entrained, and in what order, as an animal's seizure began and progressed, because that might isolate the critical structures along the route from deep brain to outer cortex. No small question. How do you watch a complex event unfold, in territory too microscopically remote to access directly? The answer was to create a series of still films that would each illuminate a key part of the causal chain.

Here is how he designed the experiment:

He would feed all the guinea pigs water laced with sugar and a radioactive compound almost identical to sugar—close enough that it would be taken up by the brain as it fed on sugar, but different enough that it would not be broken down. Radioactive, so that wherever it followed sugar in high concentration, it would leave the dark star of a radiation burn on X-ray film, indicating the intense sugar metabolism of neurons in seizure. Looking at the hundreds of photo impressions of microthin slices of frozen brain tissue, arranged front to back, Mirski would be able to spot the "sugar burst" of high metabolism demanded in the seizure nodes as neurons fired repeatedly. In effect, he was creating a kind of flip book, the predecessor of motion-picture cartoons. But Mirski would have to study each moment in the seizure painstakingly, one page at a time.

And here are the two critical controls. One guinea pig in each trial was anesthetized, nothing more. Its brain pictures would show the gray pattern of normal sugar metabolism under anesthesia. The second control was anesthetized but also got a dose of anticonvulsant drug. Its much lighter images would show the damping effect of the anticonvulsant on already-sedated metabolism.

Next, the two trial animals. One guinea pig was given a large dose of the convulsant, and its microslice photos would show dense black radiation burn in all neuron structures—bursts in the thalamus and several lower brain-stem neuron structures and, of course, over the entire cortex, the signature of a generalized seizure. Finally came the guinea pig he hoped would prove interesting. That animal was given a dose of both the convulsant and the anticonvulsant. This would be the key to the experiment, if it worked.

Begin. Inject a dose of metrazol into a guinea pig that has fed on the radioactive sugar compound. At some predetermined time, euthanize the guinea pig with an overdose of anesthetic, freezing its seizure in place, marked by the varying concentrations of radioactive sugar. Extract and freeze the brain. Slice the brain into ultrathin slivers and press each slice against an X ray plate, which will record the blackened image of a generalized seizure in progress.

And finally, most important, repeat with the animal that *could not* have a seizure, because it had been given antiseizure medication. A critical question might be answered: At what sites do those successful medications operate? They would mark the spot where the advancing seizure had been halted. If that were known, for example, and were found to be the same site in humans, a person might be given a very low dose of a powerful drug, sent right to the key brain structure, and so avoid harmful side effects.

All this was carried out in a mini–operating theater, like those here in Sherman's lab. On just such a table as Toung operated, Mirski carried out his prescribed work on the controls, then began with the experimental animals. First, he delivered precise doses of metrazol to one series of guinea pigs, then the time-stopping overdose. On to the group whose seizures would be halted. He injected doses of both the antiseizure medication that goes by the trade name Zarontin and the surefire metrazol.

When he was finished, many months later, he had created a complementary set of images, brains that were identical slice for slice except for the effects of the drugs that had coursed through them. He could put them side by side and infer the story that had unfolded. And if all went well in his analysis, he should be able to predict what would happen in a variety of circumstances.

Here is the narrative, cut to its dramatic heart—the moment of seizure, as the calm sea of the entire brain was on the verge of bursting with lightning streaks. In the animals given antiseizure drugs as well as convulsants, the glow of intense neuron firing blackened the image from the lower brain all the way to a frontal part of the thalamus—then stopped. Thanks to the medication, of course, the dark burns of seizure never went beyond that structure to the cortex. More importantly, this thalamic structure glowed hotter in the medicated animals than it did *during* full-blown seizures in the animals with no anticonvulsants.

The explanation seemed plain—at least, it was plain to Mirski. He had found the thalamic circuit that could put the brakes on some generalized brain seizures. It was located in a frontal structure of the guinea pig's thalamus. *Eureka*. How does a proven antiepileptic like Zarontin—or Depakote, or any other used against generalized seizures—succeed in preventing them? *Apparently* by powering up circuits in the anterior nucleus of the thalamus, which must be a natural counterforce against seizure. It glowed bright as he tried and failed to induce a seizure in medicated animals. It glowed, but not as bright, when unmedicated animals did have seizures, indicating that it had failed to stem the tide. The anterior nucleus truly appeared to be the action site for these major medications.

Imagine the consequences for epilepsy sufferers if Mirski were right: new drugs could be designed that would call into action only this small, deep-brain nucleus, before seizures started. No more dousing the entire brain with deadening chemicals.

Many more months down this tortuous road of experimentation, Mirski disproved his own hypothesis. In fact, he turned it on its head.

Given that the seizure-killer was a knot of neurons in the fore of the thalamus, then destroying that knot should *eliminate* the effect of anti-seizure drugs. Demonstrating this would help nail down his hypothesis. Chemically knock out the forward part of a guinea pig's thalamus, so Zarontin won't have a site to work on, give the guinea pig Zarontin, induce seizure, and you should get seizure. Simple, at least in concept. It was no mean feat to carry it out, given the structure's remoteness in the guinea pig's brain and the brain's tiny size, but he did it.

But the Zarontin-medicated animals with no frontal thalamus still failed to seize.

"The way science really works is that you do the experiment, and, instead of 'Eureka,' you come up with 'Now, isn't that peculiar?'" Mirski says.

There was one more move in this chesslike game to light up the secret, and that was to knock out that anterior nucleus of the thalamus in *un*-medicated animals. He did so, giving them metrazol but no seizure-blocker. He waited for the seizure. And waited. Soon, "peculiar" became very interesting again. Without medication, with no forward thalamus, given a dose of a never-fail convulsant, the guinea pigs did not have a seizure.

This microscopic hot zone—the anterior nucleus of the thalamus—turned out to be the *instigator* of these generalized seizures. Knock it out, and even metrazol will not induce a seizure. The thalamus's anterior nucleus must actually be disabled by drugs like Zarontin or Depakote, so that it could not amplify the brain stem signals leading to seizure. The discovery potentially was just as important to epilepsy sufferers as the one he first thought he'd made. It also made sense that this anterior pole of the thalamus was a major player in these destructive events. Much of the thalamus has specialized circuitry, such as the circuit cluster that helps turn light signals into "seeing." Such specialized circuits could not be behind generalized seizures. The anterior nucleus, in contrast, communicates with the most primitive regions of the cortex, which in turn link to all the rest.

Marek Alexander Z. Mirski, M.D., successfully defended his dissertation, *Functional Anatomy of Pentylenetetrazol Seizures,* and added Ph.D. to his academic resumé. "This thesis is dedicated to my mother and father, for their never-ending love, guidance and understanding," he wrote. "Their constant support and enthusiasm have made any problems in my life more tolerable and all of my goals easier to accomplish."

That single paragraph alludes to Mirski's two distinct "origins." The scientist has just emerged from the controlled reality of the laboratory, appropriately fluent in latinate words, words run together into tongue twisters. The son, husband, father emerged from that initial Z of his forebears, out of the same mundane, uncontrolled reality we all inhabit. These two realities have this assumption in common: Life is predictable. We rarely think about how essential this premise is to our moving forward, whether in carrying out daily routines or planning great schemes.

In Chinese, the worst curse you can hurl at a foe is this: *May you live in interesting times.* The good life is spun out of predictability. Heroic sagas arise out of chaos, and those are interesting, if you survive.

Predictable: Jerzy Zapadko, a teen-ager in Warsaw, Poland, hopes to become a doctor. The Zapadkos are strictly middle class, but with hard work his hopes are within reach. Like most of his friends, he is a member of his parish Boy Scout troop, a minor detail that will mark his life's turning point. Across town lives Janina Lutyk; she comes from a family higher in the social strata, related to the czarist Russian Romanovs on her father's side, and she has set her sights on a career in physics. Even in sophisticated Warsaw, that choice for a girl marks her as a bit of a rebel. She's a romantic rebel at that, identifying with the independent, headstrong heroine of the best-seller recently translated into Polish, *Gone With The Wind*, set in the period of America's most horrific turbulence.

Factor in the year 1939 and the predictable becomes interesting.

In September, two weeks after the Germans invade Poland from the west, starting World War II, Soviet troops march in from the east, overrunning and capturing most of the army. Sometime later, in Russia's Katyn Forest, the Soviets execute in cold blood virtually the entire Polish officer corps, more than 4,000 men. In the west, after 27 days of blitzkrieg, the Germans capture Warsaw and overrun the country. Less than two years later, they attack their Soviet allies and roll on toward Russia itself.

Jump forward those two years. Jerzy Zapadko at 17 is a leader in the Polish underground. Like many of his peers, he literally graduated from Boy Scout to Resistance fighter, although in the daylight world he is simply a student. In the absence of native civil or military authority, with most surviving soldiers either imprisoned or having fled to join Free Polish forces, the Boy Scouts have become a critical seed for the Resistance. Across town, Janina Lutyk is a student at the *gymnasium,* carrying out her studies under the eyes of the Nazi occupation. Also a Resistance member, she keeps stores of weapons and ammunition under the floorboards of her apartment, carries messages from one safe house to another, takes part in bridge demolitions. Her code name is Scarlett.

Jerzy rises to the rank of division commander in Parasol, perhaps the most famous of the Resistance groups, whose members all have a price on their heads—or on the heads of their aliases, since their identities are not known. They are the most hated by the occupiers. Parasol units sabotage tanks, artillery, and other military equipment. They assassinate Gestapo officers. At each exploit they leave their calling card with its signature open parasol, its handle an anchor. Few if any Parasol units have as long a list of scores as the division led by Jerzy Zapadko, code named Mirski. He picked the alias because it would sound like a common name to a foreigner's ear, but in fact he knew of no Mirskis in the entire country, families who might be blamed for his predations against the Nazis. A contemporary Polish account says simply, "Gestapo officer died May 22, 1943, by Mirski's action." Occasionally he and Scarlett crossed paths, but they never really got to know one another.

Jump to the summer of 1944, against which even the hellish five years before will seem orderly and serene. The Soviets, having beaten back their German invaders, march on occupied Warsaw from the east. The Allied plan calls for an uprising by Warsaw's infantry-armed Resistance, but with artillery and aircraft support from the Soviets. Once a core of the city is secured, the Polish government in exile will be flown from London to retake civilian control. On schedule, the underground Resistance blazes into the open as the Warsaw Uprising begins, and on cue the Soviets—sit on their side of the Vistula River, watch, and wait.

The Germans react with predictable ferocity, throwing tanks, artillery, and heavily armed infantry against the Resistance, slaughtering countless fighters outright and driving the encircled survivors inward from one redoubt to another. Hitler orders his commanders to destroy Warsaw, to leave neither building nor human standing. Surrounded, Jerzy Mirski and the others pour into the last escape routes—the vast underground sewers. As they flee in the darkness pursued by firing troops, soldiers above drop grenades and explosives into the tunnels, killing hundreds. The worst of it for Jerzy is having to crawl over the bodies of dead comrades as they retreat through the tunnels in a nightmare of explosions and screams. Finally they are trapped from both ends. The end seems foretold. The survivors emerge to be executed, like those captured earlier. Now, however, perhaps because German commanders sense the approaching loss of the war, they are made prisoners of war.

Across town, the Soviets finally invade and beat back the Germans—coming not as allies but as conquerors, with no more love for the Polish Resistance than the Nazis had. Janina, never taken by the Germans, now is captured by the Soviets and marched off to prison by a soldier. Her end seems equally predictable. The Russian, however, is desperate for a smoke, so he gives Janina money and sends her into a tobacco shop while he waits outside. She runs out a back door and escapes. In Italy, in a displaced persons camp, she meets again the young Parasol leader . . .

The rest, if not quite predictable, follows established pathways to achievement. Jerzy Mirski will become a Ph.D. economist in Washington, D.C. Janina Lutyk Mirski will become a civil engineer, recognized for her role in designing earthquake-proof hospitals in the United States.

THE GREEKS OBSERVED how difficult, if not impossible, prediction was. They lit on this striking anomaly as well: that it was so comparatively easy to see what the truth was, going away, looking back at it. Truth seemed to reside in the past, as though it emerged into being only as the present died.

Looking back, who cannot see the flawless, crystalline precision in every move Jerzy and Janina made within an equally clockwork world. Yet they, looking forward, had no more idea what was coming than we do of tomorrow. In fact, their knowing so well the potential consequences of their actions without a hint of what the real consequences would be is what makes them heroic. It's just that easy to trace the unambiguous origin of every force that beset them—all as clear as the path of a lightning bolt captured on fast film, its wonderful filagree burned in a pattern from sky to earth that is precisely measurable with protractor and calipers by degree of angle and millimeter of reach. But that photograph is no tool for prediction.

If you cannot predict, you do not understand. Not, at least, in this other modeling universe we have entered, which cohabits with the first. In the best of all science worlds, everything would go according to plan—it's not your plan, but you would unravel it. You would look forward and predict everything right on the money. What makes this impossible ideal doable *in part* is just that: everything must be reduced to its parts (though what constitutes a part can be tricky). You don't try to solve the world *out there*. You try to isolate tiny elements of it that you can closely observe and measure, abstracted from the whole. You tease them apart, ever more finely as need be, till you find threads whose pathways you can predict. And so on, pattern by layer by element, until you gradually assemble the parts into a model of the whole. The epic pretends to sweep forward on a grand scale, really looking backward. The scientist's experiment-story really does look forward, in tiny increments, via solid answers to small questions—the best of them, Fisher says, answerable by yes or no. Time is no obstacle.

Survival does not hang on these threads. The aim is to emerge with solid truth, testable and reliable, of "the real world." This is the realm of research—rigorous, disciplined and, above all, patient.

Jerzy and Janina kept his code name, Mirski, because they were leery of the Soviets knowing his real family name, given his ties to Parasol. Marek and his sister were born in Washington, D.C. and grew up speaking Polish "inside," where his name was pronounced with a trilled r, and speaking regular American "outside," where it's pronounced "Mark." That followed a pattern for everything spoken. "I grew up thinking it was just normal for things to have one set of names at home and another set outside," Marek Mirski says laughing. "Until I was about 10, I didn't even know I was bilingual."

Mirski's dissertation dedication moved on to Lenore, his fiancée to whom he was "forever grateful for her love and friendship." They had met in their first year of medical school, and would marry now, just before he began his internship year and she completed her residency. Another year, and they set off for Baltimore and his own residency in Johns Hopkins's Neurology Department, whose faculty included both Daniel Hanley and Robert Fisher.

HANLEY AND FISHER WERE not only colleagues and occasional collaborators, they were close friends. If Mirski's work was of interest to Hanley, who had rescued more than one near-death patient from status epilepticus, it was fundamentally important to Fisher, who was interested as an epileptologist in these action sites of the electrochemical brain. Even more to the point, Fisher was looking for ways to stop seizures by electrical stimulation. Cutting the cables between the thalamus and its forward connections, as Mirski had done on guinea pigs, would be disastrous for humans, causing catastrophic memory problems. He wanted to know if Mirski could produce the same outcome electrically as he had with the scalpel.

Working with Fisher through a series of painstaking experiments that lasted throughout his training and into his early faculty life, Mirski detailed a potential site in the thalamus for an epileptic "pacemaker." A cardiac pacemaker sets the correct beat for a heart out of rhythm. If Mirsky's device proved itself, the implant would detect aberrations emanating from the anterior thalamus and stifle them, preventing seizures from starting.

End of story? Nowhere near. This story has many very different projections, each illuminating a facet of the scientific complex into which it makes connections.

First projection. Mirski and Fisher, both M.D./Ph.D.'s, came to a critical decision at the outset of their collaboration, one that tells much of how high-stakes, first-rank science operates. Their Ph.D. side might push for a grant to precisely track the molecular chemistry of this chain reaction. That is the direction in which the National Institutes of Health has always leaned heavily in funding grant proposals. In that direction lay the rich "extramural funding" that was the lifeblood of Johns Hopkins, Harvard, Stanford—every major research institution outside the government itself. However, their M.D. training pushed them toward the electrical side of the challenge, because that would lead most quickly to patient applications. That fork in the road, molecular versus electric, indicates just how specialized research is. If the aim is to articulate the molecular mechanisms of seizure induction, go molecular. If the aim is to stem seizures in humans, go electric. Mirski and Fisher chose to study the electrical side of the problem, and it cost them. They pushed on through meager federal funding until the Epilepsy Society of America came through with support. But Fisher believes they would have added ten years to the time when there might be clinical benefit of this research had they gone in the other direction, as interesting as the questions that lay there were and are.

Projection two. Fisher left Johns Hopkins in 1993, which might have separated him from the project and ended its application to patient care. But he left for Barrow Neurological Institute, where he eventually became head of neurology, and that was a boon for their clinical hopes. Fisher soon initiated a small pilot study at Barrow, together with colleagues at the University of Pennsylvania and the University of Toronto, to implant an electrical stimulator into the thalamus of patients suffering from intractable generalized seizures. *Intractable* meant that the seizures did not respond to drug therapy. The results were good enough to extend the trial to several other centers.

Now it is being expanded into a larger clinical trial. Medtronic, the manufacturer of the device, has named Fisher to direct this pivotal trial of thalamic stimulation in people with uncontrolled seizures.

This is the very cutting edge of epilepsy research now—searching for the Holy Grail, which Fisher says is "the mechanism of epileptogenesis. How does a brain injury or a genetic predisposition lead to a lifetime of epilepsy? When we know the answer to that question—in an estimated ten to twenty years—*we will be able to prevent and cure epilepsy,* not just use drugs and devices to suppress seizures."

Meanwhile, others are pursuing different ways to intervene in the short term. A never-fail universal pacemaker. Or a pattern on a piece of graph paper that can predict, as unfailingly as Galileo's observations of Jupiter, the moment when scattered brain waves will line up in a thunderous march, then slip into a monstrous order where there should be just thrums of different harmonies emerging from millions of individual circuits. Researchers dotted across the country think they are closing in on ways to trap a seizure-in-the-making.

Two decades after Mirski began his research, he, Sherman and Wendy Ziai would present new data to the annual meeting of the epilepsy society, in hopes of sparking major funding for more widespread trials. Their new data results from studying the molecular chemistry of metrazol-induced seizures—and that's why he and Ziai were in Dave Sherman's lab today.

Projection three. *Twenty years?* After all, this was no quixotic venture. Why does it all move so slowly? Fisher, as editor-in-chief of *Epilepsia,* has a practiced, professional eye for promising research. He observed: "This has a lot to do with coordination, synergy, a lot of different impulses lining up together—and I'm not talking about seizure now but about scientific progress. There are lots and lots of interesting and important questions out there. Which ones get answered first? Which ones draw the most interest? It's very unpredictable, but it's certainly a function of what the most active people in the field are interested in themselves."

And the most active people in the field, in any field of science, are Ph.D. researchers, whose lives are dedicated to formulating and answering critical questions and who have no clinical duties or distractions. They also get no clinical salaries, so they live and die by their research funding. They most often determine the direction in which new knowledge will be found because they spend their lives in single-minded pursuit of it.

Projection four: Mirski can make a claim that few physicians or researchers can match, all the years of still inconclusive work notwithstanding. While still young, he has helped shepherd his own discovery "from bench to bedside." A fundamental bit of knowledge of scientific interest for its own sake is at the point of clinical application. Today, watching Toung, chatting with Sherman, he is off in a whole new direction, using rats now to study, indeed, the chemical signatures of seizure and the excitotoxicity associated with it.

Projection five, perhaps the most intriguing. Fisher set up the pilot trials so that each patient's "pacemaker" would be on half the time, off half the time. Neither the researcher nor the patient knew which was which at any given moment, the mark of research protocols known as double-blinded, the gold-standard of clinical trials. The timing was programmed into the device and could be monitored by a third observer. That way, wishful thinking on the part of either doctor or patient could play no role in the device's success. If the patient had a seizure when the device was turned on, only the observer would know that fact. Initial results were "mixed," Fisher recalls, but on the good side.

However, in one patient, the results were "absolutely terrific." She went from frequent, intractable seizures to none whatsoever. The result? It meant that Fisher could not ethically keep her in the trial, *because he knew the device was working.* The moment he saw that her data revealed perfect congruence—that is, when the device was on, she had no seizures, when it was off, seizures returned—he removed her from the trial. Fisher programmed her pacemaker to remain on, and she has remained seizure free in the years since. But because she did not complete the trial, Fisher had to remove her data, and that hurt the results. Therein lies one of the ironies of the controlled observation in human trials. And of course it leaves a final, gnawing question: Why was it completely successful in that one patient? Why only one?

Back in Sherman's lab, Mirski is asking the same critical question about seizure that, across the room, Bhardwaj is asking about stroke. What causes the damage? The exciting findings in the laboratory in recent decades that have translated into the clinic lead to the conclusion that the dramatic events themselves—the sudden fog of an ischemic stroke, the burst of blood in the hemorrhage victim, the flailing seizure—often cause limited damage. The real devastation comes soon after and occurs progressively, as the breakdown products of those events carrom through the brain, sparking excitatory toxicity and poisoning living cells. These events might offer places to intervene.

FOR MIRSKI, this morning's worth of pure bench science was all he would get for some time as he turned to the biggest challenge the Hopkins neurointensivists had faced during his tenure. It goes by the simple name "the Bayview commitment."

As of July 1 the neurointensivists had taken on total patient management responsibility over the eight beds in the NICU at Bayview Medical Center. The driving force of that commitment was necessity. Control had become so bad at Bayview, Mirski says flatly, that the nurses were threatening to quit—threatening very seriously—and experienced nurses are the sentinels of any unit's health, all the more so an intensive care unit's health. Fisher had said years earlier, "Any young intensive-care doctor who ignores an experienced neuro nurse's warnings is headed for big trouble. They're the eyes and ears of the unit."

Bayview was mired in trouble. Alessandro Olivi, who is a professor of neurosurgery at Johns Hopkins Hospital but directs neurosurgery at Bayview, had pressed for the neurointensivists to take over. Both the retired and current chairs of neurosurgery were one hundred percent behind them. This was not a task to be undertaken lightly, however, because any problems running the NICU at Bayview, even if inherited, would now be the neurointensivists' responsibility—meaning, utlimately, Mirski's.

But he had made the commitment gladly, for his own reasons. It was another opportunity to show what trained neurointensivists could do. "You always want to go first," Mirski says. "Then you become the template for what comes later."

CHAPTER 7

Out of the Blue

Bayview Medical Center

Baltimore

July 5

THE NEUROSCIENCES conference room at Bayview looks out from a hillside over the east Baltimore neighborhood. The medical center originally served as a community hospital. This morning the air is crackling clear, the thunderstorms of the Fourth having washed it clean and left it dry. The view is stunning, for Bayview is aptly named, perched high over the Chesapeake. Johns Hopkins took over the troubled hospital in 1983, but, until a few years ago, did not have the staff to cover more than emergency neurosurgery. That meant that patients with life-threatening neurological problems had to be taken to Johns Hopkins Hospital instead of here. In this first month of "the Bayview commitment," Mirski had pledged to maintain the NICU at the same high level as downtown, allowing Bayview to accept such neurosurgery patients. Early on this fifth day of the new order, a helicopter roared in with the first out-of-area neuro emergency: Rita Serianni, 56, with symptoms of a hemorrhagic stroke.

"WHAT WILL GET YOUR ATTENTION *every time?*" Romer Geocadin asks the Bayview residents, some in their first week of neurology or neurosurgery training, others entering a new year. And he picks from the scattered answers the one for focus today: "Change in mental status, yes." A patient goes from perfectly alert and in excruciating pain to fuzzy uncertainty about what brought her here. A common emergency in the NICU. And at the far end of change in mental status? "Coma."

The helicopter had lifted into the dark, clearing sky after 4 a.m. carrying Phil and Rita Serianni from one stage of rescue to the next. Her head was splitting, she told him. He comforted her the best he could, frightened but not letting on. He would reflect on the previous night often this month. *Nothing was out of the ordinary. It was the Fourth of July. We had dinner about 7. We were planning to go to the fireworks but they were rained out, so we watched TV and, about 11 or so, I went upstairs to the bathroom to get ready for bed. All of a sudden I heard Rita cry out, in pain. I ran down. She was on the floor and trying to get up, but she couldn't. I helped her. Then I called 911 and they took her to Howard County.*

Geocadin got the page at 4 a.m. They saw Rita on rounds this morning as she lay talking with her husband, who bent over her, stroking her arm. A few minutes later she began drifting. Now she was comatose.

Stroke? Very possibly, and if not already, then potentially soon. From her symptoms, it seemed likely she had an aneurysm begin to bleed, as dangerous as any event in the brain but not necessarily fatal to brain tissue at once. Caustic blood normally kept from the delicate neurons by the blood-brain barrier now bathed them, at least in the hemorrhage area, like a corner of a growing field flooded over. Stroke is the most common emergency they treat, and its treatment as an emergency, as a brain at-tack on the level of a heart attack, was considered a real victory for the in-tensivist approach to the brain.

Every year nearly 750,000 Americans suffer strokes, and about 80 percent survive. Those sound like good odds, until you consider that two thirds of the survivors suffer some degree of disability—that means nearly 400,000 people a year. Yet until a few years ago physicians routinely did nothing to treat most strokes, on the grounds that there was nothing to do. They made the patient comfortable and hoped for the best. *Nothing* is the key word, and its Latin equivalent, *nihil,* becomes *nihilist,* the label neu-rointensivists and stroke specialists use most often to describe those who favor a hands-off approach to treating symptoms of what could become cere-bral infarction.

So the topics for this morning's whiteboard talk in the Bayview NICU conference room were chosen, as often, not from a pre-set curriculum for the new hospital year—that was for the early years of medical school—but by the helicopter flying in or ambulance rolling up to the ER door. There were two roads into the NICU, the emergency room and the oper-ating room. They were ready and waiting for those from the OR. For the emergency transfers they had to be ready for anything. In Rita Serianni's case, they would get both ER and OR, in succession.

"The two most common causes of coma that we see? Subarachnoid hemorrhage and hydrocephalus." The first a bleeding into the brain, usu-ally from an artery, the second a buildup of water pressure that must be checked. Either can be fatal or disabling, but the hemorrhage is more dan-gerous, and dangerous more quickly. Hydrocephalus is more common, and the quickest way to relieve it is by inserting an intraventricular catheter. That will drain cerebrospinal fluid and make room for the extra water. But if the problem is caused in whole or in part by an aneurysm, then reducing that pressure could allow it to rupture.

Subarachnoid hemorrhage—SAH—has nearly the highest mortality of any brain injury. One of its most dangeous causes is an aneurysm, which might go from leaking blood to rupturing outright. Despite the development of ever-better techniques for treating aneurysms over the past generation, large numbers of the victims of rupture never make it to treatment because they either die en route or cannot be resuscitated on arrival.

So what to do if hydrocephalus is suspected? "Go ahead and catheterize, but set the valve to a high pop-off." In other words, set the escape valve to allow a tolerable amount of pressure to build within the brain, enough to hold an aneurysm intact, not enough to crush brain tissue; if too much pressure builds up, the valve will pop and release the excess. The endless balancing act.

Nevertheless, an aneurysm was what Geocadin believed Serianni had suffered, a leakage of blood into her brain, and that was soon confirmed by an angiogram. An aneurysm swells like the weak point in a tire tube or balloon, the vessel wall stretching membrane-thin and eventually becoming porous enough for blood to leak through it. Luckily, Rita was already in the aneurysm survivor group; hers had only bled. But even in that survivor group, the death of brain tissue from loss of blood supply—stroke—eventually kills a large number of patients or leaves them vegetative. Still, two major changes in recent years had been improving those odds. Emergency specialists were recognizing stroke symptoms and getting victims to specialized units like this within the so-called "golden hour" when permanent deficits could be avoided. Second, treatments for the aneurysms that could lead to hemorrhagic strokes were being revolutionized by development of coiling—used to treat Michael Sanders at Columbia—as well as by better techniques of neurosurgery to deal with those whose bulbous swellings had to be clipped. Both methods were aimed at preventing outright rupture, for rupture of a major artery in the brain usually means instant death.

The neurosurgical protocols for treating aneurysms had changed dramatically over two decades. Columbia neurosurgery director Robert Solomon remembers caring for patients as a resident for up to ten days before neurosurgeons would operate on them. As a young attending neurosurgeon, he became part of the movement, spearheaded at Columbia and several other major institutions, to operate almost immediately to clip aneurysms. Why the change? Or rather, why the former ten-day wait? The belief that waiting before surgery improved survival odds was based on flawed data, Solomon recalled. How America's best brain doctors came to rely on flawed data offers a dramatic illustration of the kinds of tricks of nature even the most scrupulous researchers face. Visual certainty fades in twilight, which often confers the illusion of certainty in its place, because you can't see everything that's there. Similarly, bad data can emerge from good efforts because critical elements of the data do not show. In their professional jargon, medical researchers talk about taking the mountains of statistics on individual patients collected by thousands of physicians and "drilling out" the relevant data from the giant databases. It's an apt image, like drilling for oil with a hollow drill that will pull out the perfect core gleaming with black gold. Eureka! But to continue the analogy, do you drill *here* or *there*? Straight down or at an angle? If there were one true method of data analysis that would always reveal the clearest portrayal of reality, no one would argue over protocols—or, for that matter, the economy.

Here is how neurosurgeons were misled by apparently good numbers. Twenty-five years ago, few techniques had been developed for intensive care of the injured brain in preparation for surgery. For a variety of reasons, some patients were operated on for aneurysms quickly, others a few days later, still others many days after admission to the hospital. The surgery itself was more dangerous than it is today; far fewer patients "came out as they went in," as the medical saying puts it. Data painstakingly gathered around the world over a period of years showed that those operated on quickly did uniformly worse than those operated on after a wait of days in the hospital—and the longer the wait, the better the patients did, up to ten days after the event that hospitalized them. There was a plausible explanation: Resting, the delayed patients had stabilized over time, building up strength for the ordeal of general anesthesia and neurosurgery. It was plausible, but wrong.

When finally studied from a different angle, the data revealed another secret: huge numbers of the delayed-surgery patients died before they could reach the operating room. Thus, they did not show up on the morbidity and mortality statistics of neurosurgery. Those who survived the ten days stable enough for surgery probably were not nearly as sick to begin with as those who died—also plausible. The earlier analysts had been comparing two very different groups, without knowing it. The "immediate surgery" group included the whole gamut of aneurysm patients, from most to least serious; the "delayed surgery" group included only those well enough to have hung on for ten days.

The bottom line? Intensive care methods had to be developed to put patients in the best possible condition for neurosurgery, as quickly as they could be stabilized. That was just what Alex Olivi had pressed for here at Bayview, preoperative care that would stabilize his patients before the shock of neurosurgery, then ease them out of danger postoperatively.

Only with the neurointensive team in place could aneurysm surgery be performed here.

As Geocadin drew a snaking artery on the marker board, inked in the bulge of an aneurysm, and listed the potential complications of its bleeding, they talked over the treatments needed to hold Rita Serianni in place until Olivi could operate.

All they knew so far from the CT scans was that she had suffered a hemorrhage. As Geocadin put it, they had to answer the "chicken and egg" question: Did Rita fall and fracture her skull, causing the hemorrhage, or did she suffer the hemorrhage for another reason, causing her to fall? An MRI answered the question: there was the aneurysm, puffed out on the right anterior cerebral artery.

Initially it had seemed possible that she might be a candidate for coiling. That procedure is far less risky in itself than neurosurgery because it is non-invasive—the coil payload is inserted through a catheter in the major thigh artery and guided delicately into place in the brain. However, it was still not clear—again from that worldwide data—that *over the long term* a coil balled up inside the aneurysm bulb is as successful as a clip that pinches off the weakened bulb from the rest of the artery. But as soon as the scans had arrived in radiology, it became clear to Geocadin and the other attendings gathered around that, for Rita, it had to be surgery. The neck of her aneurysm was too wide to hold a coil. And this was going to be a tough neurosurgery. That was equally clear. From the first scans, there was something unusual about this one, and unusual is hardly ever good.

That Olivi, a Johns Hopkins neurosurgeon, could operate on such a dangerously ill patient here at Bayview, rather than having to take her downtown, was a first measure of the neurointensivists' newly expanded service. Nothing had changed in the OR since July 1. What had changed was the specialty care Serianni would receive once she passed through the doors into the NICU.

The neurosurgeon and neurologist are in many ways opposite personalities drawn together by a common obsession—an obsession with "neuro," the brain. Neurosurgeons study brain scans of every type available, picturing in their minds what these projections of the three-dimensional brain will look like close at hand, in light brighter than day. That is their defining moment: *there is the brain,* and they have to deal with it. Neurosurgery is a specialty only a century old. For half that time, in terrain where major structures are measured in millimeters and crucial vessels are the size of a hair, its morbidity and mortality were so high that truly elective neurosurgery was rare. The introduction of the intraoperative microscope in the 1960s began a revolution that empowered those with the skills and the patience and fortitude to use them. The only way to appreciate the difficulty of that job—other than spending seven years in residency learning it—is to watch it up close, often.

Neurosurgery requires an intensity of focus over many hours that is perhaps unmatched in medicine, where focus is always critical. Yet neurosurgeons live to operate. Rafael Tamargo, a top vascular neurosurgeon, had been dismayed for years by the number of elective patients who had to be turned away from Johns Hopkins to find other hospitals, for lack of NICU beds to support their neurosurgeries. "Last year we had 58 turnbacks," he said to Mirski one day recently. The pain of those lost elective cases—*lost rescues*—was palpable in someone like Tamargo, ordinarily full of good humor and optimism. Neurosurgeons may run the gamut in terms of good humor or lack of it, but optimism is a defining trait. If healing could be willed by faith and positive thinking, neurosurgery would have no bad outcomes. With the expansion of the NICU, the neurosurgeons were hoping for no turn-backs. The terrain that vascular neurosurgeons dwell in is as complex as any known, even relative to other areas of neurosurgery. As for faith and optimism, Alex Olivi would turn out needing all that he could muster this afternoon.

But the neurosurgeon's ability to see, touch, and fix the brain as an object in space also illuminates just how hard the neurologist's job is. Neurologists' defining actions start today, as centuries ago, when a patient presents with symptoms that their experience tells them can be traced into the brain. The neurologist observes, ponders, hypothesizes—then studies all the most-modern scans as ardently as the surgeon, for confirmation or rejection, for nuance and detail—for conclusion, if possible. Nevertheless, you will hear many of the neurology attendings here in intensive care remind fellows and residents that no scan can replace "the neurological exam." It is the neurologist's trademark, an entire program of examination of physical responses to questions, to touches, movements, probes so subtle in what they tell the experienced practitioner that the neuro exam reveals deficits hours or days before they become visible on any scan. What is the point of predicting the future? To alter it.

Here, for now, is the ultimate scan: Read millions of bits of information coming out of this sealed dome and deduce from them what is going on inside. Then figure from that reading what will happen; take steps to prevent the bad and enhance the good—all without literally going in there.

No two approaches to the same terrain could be more different. An adage has it that neurologists learn brain function stroke by stroke; that over time they learn, through the deficits and recoveries of patients with localized brain death through loss of similarly localized blood supply, to give their own meanings to the place-names on anatomical charts. Neurosurgeons work the geography of that terrain in perfect complement, rivers and streams, hills and valleys, cables of nerve endings laid open be-

fore them. Hands off, hands on. And now, standing between these approaches, the neurointensivist. Always hands on, always from outside.

THE MAJOR ARTERIAL LANDMARK at the core of the human
brain is a complex structure called the circle of Willis. Because of the size
of the arteries that make up the circle and the power of the blood coursing through them, they are common sites of aneurysms and hemorrhage;
because of their importance in delivering blood to the brain, these arteries are the most dangerous sites. The structure was first correctly described in both form and function in 1664 by Thomas Willis, and his is
one of those major achievements in which theory and observation must
meet in synergy before the truth can emerge. The individual arteries, after all, had been seen by dissectors since ancient times, and everyone
knew that when they were cut, blood spurted out of them. But until William
Harvey established the *circulation* of the blood and the meaning of that
to the function of organs, the importance and relationship of those arteries could not be understood. Earlier efforts had been like trying to understand an electric wiring network without knowing what electricity does.
But Willis's success also owes to another gift of the Renaissance: the ability to visualize complexity. Willis's description of the form and function of
the circle was published with illustrations by the great architect and designer
Christopher Wren.

To the untutored eye, what the structure most resembles when seen
at autopsy is a tangle of yarn, whose ropes begin on the underside of the
brain and spread upward into its lobes. Dissected out, as Willis did, they
resemble the criss-crossing web on a loom. Only if you see how blood can
flow among the arteries does the circle emerge in a pattern that must be
called ingenious—whether the emergent genius of natural selection or
the innate genius of design is moot. The circle is fed from below by the four

large arteries that supply the brain with all of its blood. First, the left and right internal carotid arteries climb the sides of the neck straight from the heart, leading into this traffic circle from below, on the left and right. At the rear, the left and right vertebral arteries run up the front of the spinal cord, then merge to form the basilar artery, which joins the circle of Willis posteriorly. Three roads in, many roads out of the circle, paired left and right: anterior cerebral arteries, middle cerebral arteries, posterior . . . and so forth. And a neuro specialist can assign a relative importance to each of these pairs, determined by which brain structures they keep alive with sugar and oxygen. Number one in importance is the singular basilar artery, which invests the brain stem. The brain stem controls heartbeat, breathing, and other automatic functions without which death is immediate. Forwardmost, the anterior cerebral arteries supply motor controls for muscles, including those for the lower limbs.

To get a sense of the multiple dimensions in which the circle nests, hold your two hands up, wrists and thumbs touching, as though raising up a chalice—or the circle of Willis. Looking at the brain from the rear, your thumbs would brush the vertebral arteries, and the basilar would run above and between them. Your pinkies would follow the anterior cerebral arteries. All of the arteries splay outward, down, up, investing the entire upper brain with blood. Two "communicating arteries" complete the circle by linking its left and right sides—anteriorly and posteriorly. They are called A-comm and P-comm for short. The critical point is not that blood flows around the circle— normally it does not. The critical point is that in a crisis, it can. Like many systems, especially within the brain, this offers protection against failure. If one artery becomes slowly occluded, others can gradually enlarge in response, so that blood delivered for one side of the brain eventually can be shared by both. Sometimes, even the sudden blocking of an artery on one side, say, by a clot, can be offset by collateral flow from the opposite side.

This was the terrain that Olivi would have to reach today, at the base of the skull, itself the most difficult place to get to and in which to work. As Geocadin and the residents examined Serianni's scans, they could see the bulge of the aneurysm just at the front of the right anterior cerebral artery, at the front of the circle of Willis. The complication they had seen was that the aneurysm appeared to be dual-lobed—that is, the arterial weakness had caused the vessel to send out two balloons in different planes. And that was only what they could see.

IT WAS NOW AFTERNOON on a day turned windy and threatening more rain. Phil Serianni had been up all night, having arrived with his wife, and by now he had been joined by their daughter Monica, 21. Natalie, 25, and Suzanne, 23, were on their way. They are an athletic family. All three girls were standouts in soccer and Phil played semi-professional football well enough to spend much of his time in the army playing football. Rita had been in good health, an active, on-the-go woman who worked part-time and spent much of the rest of her day in neighborhood activities. "Yesterday she spent most of the day shopping to get ready for a neighbor's wedding shower she was putting on," Phil said. "That's her, she's always doing things like that." She'd had no warning signs, although she was being treated for hypertension. That is a risk factor for aneurysms. She smokes, another risk factor for aneurysms and a major one for women, for reasons not known. Dr. Geocadin, who had explained the situation to him earlier, now went through the trials that lay ahead.

"I'm a neurointensivist. That means I will take care of things right up to the surgery and come back to her right after," he said. "You're in the hands of the best team for this. We will give her the best chance." Geocadin was optimistic but pulled no punches. There would be two parts to bringing her back, each with its own set of risks. There was the neurosurgery, and its risks would be immediate. Death, of course, was number one. But there were risks that the aneurysm could rebleed as the pressure of the surrounding brain was relieved, and that could cause a full-blown stroke. The good news was that stroke probably had not occurred yet. Rita probably had not permanently lost any brain function. There were also risks in the anesthesia that would be needed for the surgery.

Then there would be part two, risks postop. Phil tucked the information away. First things first. It had been a long day already by the time Rita was wheeled from the unit down the hall to neurosurgery; now, just past noon, it would draw longer and grow tense as the Seriannis sat in the family waiting room.

V o i c e s   b e h i n d   m a s k s : "Is she ready for the OR?"

"Vitals are okay."

"Type and cross two units of blood."

Now she crosses over, through the wide door of the OR.

O l i v i   s c r u b s   i n   as the patient is being swathed head to foot in sheets and sterile toweling, leaving only a small area exposed for the operation. He and two assisting residents study her scans on the wall. Eric Amundson, the chief resident, will open and close. Olivi will use a right temporal approach. Amundson shaves her scalp on the right front quadrant, and with a purple felt marker draws a semicircle from just above the eyebrows, dead center, arcing across her forehead to just in front of the right ear, ending at the temple. A straight line connecting the arch completes the trace of the skin flap to be tacked back and of the underlying bone flap to be removed.

At 1:30, as the operation is about to start, the blood bank calls. There has been an "oversight." The patient's name was misspelled at some stage in the registration process, and the blood sample needed to bring up two units of the right blood type, to hold in case needed for transfusion, has been lost. They need another sample. Scrub nurse and anesthesiologist are plainly angry. This means a delay. They send down another blood sample.

Scans show blood in the fourth ventricle, the lowest of the cerebrospinal fluid cisterns, right behind the brain stem. And the lateral horns of both left and right ventricles are enlarged; they are the uppermost and by far the largest cisterns, with arms filling in large hollows between the left and right frontal lobes and the temporal lobes. To the practiced eye, the shape of the swollen upper ventricles suggests that the origin of the blood was from either the right anterior cerebral artery or A-comm, which links the right to the left. Now they can see that the two aneurysm bulbs are indeed on the anterior cerebral artery.

Downtown—at Johns Hopkins Hospital—a study is underway comparing coiling versus clipping, specifically for aneurysms of the anterior cerebral arteries and of A-comm. Johns Hopkins is the only U.S. participant in this randomized coil/clip trial, which is part of a large European study. Patients who are enlisted in the study are selected randomly for one or the other. For once, the study is large enough and has been going on long enough that its investigators hope to learn if one method is truly superior to the other procedure. This is the kind of study whose outcome could quickly change the practice of neurological medicine around the world. With Phil Serianni's consent, Rita has already been enrolled in one clinical trial, testing whether a patient's being cooled during surgery improves outcome.

Now an OR team member raises the importance of the coil-versus-clip trial. "Is there no chance of getting her into the study?" one of the on-lookers asks.

"No chance," Olivi says in the Italian accent of his native Padua. "There are two lobes here that I can see, and neither has a neck." It would be the neck of the puffed-out aneurysm that would have to hold the twisted coil in place within the bulb of the aneurysm. The lack of that neck will complicate Olivi's clipping job as well. "This is a bad, nasty aneurysm," he says, half to himself. From a neurosurgeon's view, the anterior communicating artery is harder to reach and to work around than some others, though the toughest is agreed to be the basilar tip, at the rear of the circle of Willis. But location is only part of what makes clipping an aneurysm difficult. Shape plays a major role, and this one is a monster, twin-lobed and irregular. Olivi stares thoughtfully at the scans on the wall one last time before starting and repeats, "Nasty. Very nasty."

Gino Vista and Sandy Osborn, taping electrical leads to the patient's scalp, are specialists in operating the evoked potential monitor. Evoked potential monitoring is one of the most important advances in brain protection during neurosurgery, taking advantage of the brain's electrical nature in a deceptively simple way. Deceptive, because years of clinical trials were necessary to refine it as a useful tool. Each anterior cerebral artery feeds the part of the motor cortex that controls movement of the leg on the opposite side. The aneurysm is on the right, so it is the brain's continued ability to control the left leg that they want to watch, as a guarantee that that brain region is still receiving enough blood. Thus, throughout the surgery, Vista and Osborn will send electric pulses to Serianni's right motor strip, and they will watch for slight responsive movements of her left leg beneath the blankets.

Olivi considers his approach. He will have to lift up the frontal lobe and push onward, below it and above the resting temporal lobe. "I need to position the head so that gravity helps lift the brain gently," he says, adjusting the clamp holding her head in place. When he can see the optic nerve heading toward the rear of the brain from the right eye, he will bring in the intraoperative microscope. "The problem is that because of the recent bleed the anatomy is distorted by blood," he says.

Resident: "Are you concerned about a rebleed as you expose the aneurysm?"

"Absolutely. And the aneurysm could rupture on its own at any time." That could be fatal in an artery of that size unless the bleeding is quickly controlled. At work now, positioned over the patient, he says to the questioning resident, "Come to my left. I want you to see what I do."

IT IS 3:30 WHEN THE ANSPACH BONE saw whines, the bone flap is quickly removed, and the dura is exposed for the first time in this patient's life to the air—though fortunately to the high-filtered air of the operating room. Filtered or not, airborne infection remains a postoperative risk. It also could slip in here, in the brush of an unsterile towel, something the nurses are ever on the alert for, especially when there are visitors in the OR. It could come more easily as the patient lies through a long recovery, the sutured wound still open to penetration by a microbe. Olivi and Amundson now work wearing headpieces of fiber-optic cables that glow an eerie blue and send two bright, tight beams of light onto the exposed brain. The dura is retracted and they stare into the gap between temporal and frontal lobes called the Sylvian sulcus—Latin for the fissure of Sylvius. There is the optic nerve. In comes the Leica intraoperative microscope.

Soon they see the aneurysm. "That's the easy part done," Olivi says, backing out momentarily as he asks for 10 cc's of cerebrospinal fluid to be drawn off, to relax the brain tissue and make the view more open. "If only the field were more dry," he says, back at it. He is in dangerous territory now, with the brain exposed and retracted and the field blurred by fluid. They suction, they irrigate, they suction, he probes.

At 4:55, good news: the leg evokes look good. The right brain's ability to control the left leg movement is apparently unhindered. No stroke, so far.

For more than half an hour Olivi works simply to expose the aneurysm and clear blood from the field. His voice calm, then exasperatedly complaining to no one, then calm; emotion all bound up in the voice. To watch him almost motionless at work, it appears the audio track has been mismatched to the video; there is no body language corresponding to the voice. The hands delicately probe; the voice complains. What an impossible aneurysm. What difficult terrain.

Finally, very bad news: "There are two entirely different aneurysms here. I have to isolate the big one, but then I will have to be ready because there will not be much time to get the small one." It is the large one that is double-lobed, shaped like a sausage pinched at the center as it swells from the joint of the anterior cerebral and A-comm arteries. Tough as it is, he seats the clip in one try on the large aneurysm, but the small one is a devil. "I'm losing it! Losing it! Lost it!" The smaller bulb will not hold the clip.

He asks the evokes tech, "Gino, any changes?"

"So far we're looking good, Dr. O," Vista replies.

At 5:30 he calls Radiology for an angiogram, to check cerebral blood flow and make sure he is not causing stroke along any of the neighboring arteries of the circle of Willis.

Frequently he asks, "How we doing, Gino?"

Always gets, "Looks good, Dr. O, no changes."

There are a dozen different shapes of aneurysm clips available to him, and Olivi tries several before settling on one that is fenestrated—the opening of the clip is in the center, rather than at the end, so it will in effect strangle off the dome of the small aneurysm. "I am still fighting for control," he says.

It soon becomes apparent that he can control the aneurysm only by clipping off the right anterior cerebral artery, permanently closing off its blood supply. Loss of such a major vessel in the circle of Willis could send shock waves of infarction throughout its territory, but the certain rupture of the aneurysm if not bypassed would be fatal. On the other hand, if the collateral blood flow that is the evolutionary function of the circle of Willis is strong enough, there might be relatively little long-term impact. He looks at the scans again, considers the options, which continually narrow to one. Sacrifice the artery.

Finally, just after six o'clock, he manages to tie off the smaller dome. He is troubled by having to clip off such an artery to do so. But the news from the evoked potential monitor is better than good. "There must be very strong collateral flow," Olivi says, "because there is no change in the evokes." Blood from the corresponding arteries on the left is making up for that lost on the right. So far, so good.

"Tell the family the aneurysm is clipped and we're doing an intraoperative angiogram," he says. "Scope out." This is the moment the tension breaks in neurosurgery. Nothing left but to close. But it is after 7 before closing begins, when Olivi is convinced from the angiogram and scans that there is nothing more to be done today, so he leaves the stitching to his chief resident and bends over his operating notes to complete the report.

He and the anesthesiologist are exiting the OR into the window-lined hallway just after 7, and suddenly the heavens open up. Rain in sheets drives and slashes against the tall windows. The wind is banging at the windows and tall trees can be seen heaving and bending beyond. No ordinary thunderstorm. In fact, right now, the news later will report, a tornado is touching down in nearby Woodlawn.

The physicians appear oblivious. Olivi replays the case. "I took out two separate aneurysms" at the the place where the bridging anterior communicating artery joins with the right anterior cerebral. But "I had to sacrifice the right. There were two lobes on just one of the aneurysms and it would not tie off." A crucial artery to sacrifice, he says again, but the news from the evoked potentials remained good. He continues, "We preserved performance in the dominant hemisphere. Every move we made was a move of no return."

"We have flow, we've got flow" throughout the brain, the anesthesiologist replies, congratulating Olivi: "Such a bad presentation!" Then he adds, "We're going to get a jump on vasospasm" by keeping Serianni's medication high.

"There are two parts to this game," Geocadin had told Phil Serianni. "The surgery is the first half. But there is a whole second half, and it is in the second half that the neurointensivist plays the vital role." They would face three primary risks. "Vasospasm begins five to seven days out and begins to shut down arteries; we don't know why. But it can lead to ischemic stroke. Next, we have to be on guard against hydrocephalus, water entering the brain tissue that causes swelling." And finally, they would have to deal with edema, a swelling of the brain tissue itself that comes days after surgery. Geocadin explained that the effect of edema is "just like after you bang your arm. You feel a lot of pain from the damaged tissue, but it's not swollen. The swelling comes days later." External tissue, of course, is free to swell without hindrance, so a swollen arm is only an annoyance. Swelling of the brain against the skull can destroy it.

Luck

Johns Hopkins Hospital

July 13

ALL THOSE who arrive from a trauma scene today can swear to this: bad luck struck on Friday the thirteenth. But luck is tricky because, like everything, it is many layered, and as you pump up the resolution on your unlucky thirteenth, you may find a whole different take on things nesting inside. Maybe this was your lucky day in the end.

OUT THE DOOR of the NICU goes Trina Cunningham all in a rush, her yellow, throw-away OR gown streaming behind as she writes on a clipboard. Cunningham, an RN, developed an interest in research several years ago and now carries out much of the coordination and legwork for several clinical trials underway in neuro critical care. She catches up with and follows the gurney bearing Donna Soja, a 28-year-old mother of three about to undergo craniotomy to have an aneurysm clipped, just as Rita Serianni did on an earlier day. Cunningham hopes to enroll Soja in a clinical trial, called by its easily remembered acronym, IHAST2.

Of the hundreds of clinical trials going at Johns Hopkins at this moment, few make it so clear that those who try to heal the brain work in a world where uncertainty is too often unmeasurable. That is a limit to science, whether "applied," as in medicine, or in the most "basic" molecular biology. Science rarely, if ever, achieves certainty. Even early consensus is unusual; dispute is the order of the day. One hallmark of science, however, is the drive to measure how uncertain you are of what you know. For example, when driving in fog, you know you are not seeing clearly, but if you can clearly make out just the shapes of objects 200 yards up the road, then you have a good idea of what you can and cannot see. That can be a difference between tolerable and fatal uncertainty.

For years, many of those who operate deep in the brain—so far nearly always necessary when pursuing aneurysms of major arteries, such as those emanating from the circle of Willis—have followed the evidence that cold is protective of the brain. And the evidence is good, as far as it goes. The limiting case offers an example. There is a procedure of anesthesia, called "standstill" for short, that is both chilling and numbing. It has been performed successfully with any frequency at only two medical centers in the United States, Barrow Neurological Institute in Phoenix, where more than 100 procedures have been conducted, and Columbia, which has completed 65. The standstill brings patients slowly down from body temperature to below room temperature—between 60 and 65 degrees Fahrenheit. They are not only anesthetized but in barbiturate coma. At this point, with brain metabolism so unmeasurably low that neurons are not firing at all, the patient's blood is drained into a circulating machine that keeps it from coagulating. In this state, as close to suspended animation as humans have ever come and lived, neurosurgeons can clip off deep brain aneurysms with the operating field clear of blood and with inner brain structures more accessible and malleable. Barrow researchers not only have gathered voluminous evidence that such hypothermia—low temperature—is protective, they have measured variations in protection over a range of temperatures. It seems a clear case where science and intuition fit hand in glove. We've all read of near drownings from which victims recovered because they were in near-freezing water, and we all know that our chilled extremities lose feeling—become anesthetized. Most of the 100 Barrow standstill patients had the most-dangerous basilar tip aneurysms and were operated on by director Robert Spetzler, and most of them recovered completely.

As a result of evidence like this, many neurosurgeons routinely operate on aneurysms after chilling patients somewhat. Not to the dramatic degree of the standstill, which requires a highly trained, coordinated team of surgical and nursing specialists and technicians, but in the low 90 degrees Fahrenheit range. Does this help protect the brain and thus improve outcome? That is precisely what IHAST2 aims to measure.

Intraoperative Hypothermia for Aneurysm Surgery Trial #2: one randomly selected group of patients is operated on under hypothermic conditions, their bodies chilled to 91.4 degrees Fahrenheit by having cold water pumped into the mattresses under them; a second randomly selected group is operated on at normal OR temperature. The patients are selected randomly, however, only after they have met strict eligibility criteria, and one of those criteria seems odd. Only patients headed for surgery whose aneurysms have already bled may be considered for hypothermia. Why so? Because the pilot study (IHAST1), which included *any* patient undergoing aneurysm surgery, showed a possible, small benefit only to those whose aneurysms had already bled, and no benefit to the others. (And, most important of course, no harm to any of them.)

When this new worldwide trial on 900 patients has been completed, the results will be studied. This study is double-blind. That means that neither the patient nor the neurosurgeon knows which protocol is in effect, which has led to more than a few OR cracks. "You mean you can't tell if your patient is frozen or not?" And has led to a question for the neurosurgeon on Trina Cunningham's clipboard: Do you think your patient in this case was or was not in a condition of hypothermia? Among the data researchers will slice and dice will be the accuracy of the surgeons' responses. Early data indicate that they are right only about half the time— that is, their answers are in the accuracy range of random guesses, just as researchers would hope. (Technically, this protocol is considered only "partial blinded," because the anesthesia half of the operating team is responsible for controlling the patient's temperature, and there could be no guessing on their part.)

DONNA SOJA WAS SITTING on her front steps near Dover, Delaware, yesterday, off and on, enjoying a cigarette and keeping an eye on her three boys, ages 6, 8 and 9, as they played. After lunch she took them over to her mother's house. She and her mother chatted in between Donna's spells with the kids outside. In the early evening, Donna was outside talking to a neighbor; she came in to tell her mother she had a stiff neck. Pressure was building. No headache at first, just that strange feeling of pressure. "You know how it is when you're coming down on an airplane and your ears pop?" she said. "Something like that." Then her vision started to blur. Sit down, her mother, Cheri Cox, told her. Take it easy. Donna called in to the Hardee's where she works evenings as a shift leader and said she was ill. Then she crossed the floor toward her mother, and her knees buckled. Cheri called the family doctor, who thought this was a migraine attack. But it felt nothing like a migraine to Donna, who had suffered them most of her life, and a few minutes later her mother followed her instincts and punched 911. Within an hour of that stiff neck, Donna was at Kent Hospital. Her husband, John, left as early as he could from his night-shift shipping job, and he met them at the hospital.

It was after two in the morning when Donna was loaded onto a helicopter. There was the stomach-churning sway of its lifting, the noise. Now she looks up at a circle of faces over hers, just inside the OR doors at Johns Hopkins Hospital, a little before noon on Friday.

Neurosurgeon Daniele Rigamonti looks in on the circle and talks to Donna. After a while he leaves for lunch, the only break he will take until evening, after he has scrubbed out and left Ronald Clatterbuck to close. Clatterbuck just completed his final, chief resident year on June 30 and stayed on as a new assistant professor while contemplating continuing with a fellowship somewhere. An anesthesia resident who has been talking to Cunningham is explaining the controlled trial on hypothermia that is taking place. Soja "is randomized to hypothermia or no-hypothermia, but you won't know which," the resident tells Clatterbuck. "I'm supposed to ask you if you can tell." He says, "Won't I just see the [temperature] numbers on the monitor?" "No, I have to cover them up," she replies. The anesthesia team members must know which protocol is being followed, because it is they who will pump either chilled or neutral-temperature water into the cooling mattress on which Soja will lie.

Rigamonti, like Olivi, is Italian, hailing from the city of Pergamo, north of Milan. Over lunch he reflects on the upcoming clipping of Donna Soja's aneurysm. "I've seen much worse," he says. But he recalls when he was starting out and had the good fortune to work alongside Dr. Gazi Yasargil, the Turkish-born neurosurgeon who had pioneered the new world of mi-croneurosurgery in the mid-1960s. "I asked him, 'After so many thou-sands of aneurysm surgeries, what can you tell me, a young guy, to ease the tension before surgery begins?' And he said, 'I'll tell you that after many thousands of aneuryms a simple one can go wrong. And if it goes wrong, the patient dies. My heart never goes down until the clip is on.' " So much for easing the tension.

Remembering that the two halves of the circle of Willis are visually completed by two communicating arteries makes Soja's surgery easy to pic-ture. Serianni's aneurysms included the anterior communicating artery, A-comm. Soja's is on the posterior communicating artery, P-comm.

Soja has just given Cunningham her informed consent to be part of the IHAST2 study. And before that she and John had signed all the in-formed consent papers for her neurosurgery. Risks of neurosurgery in-clude death. Understand? Yes. All that had been drawn out more slowly and carefully, of course, but there it was. Donna has been here before, in a sense, and it's hard for her to tell if that makes it better or worse. When she was 10, riding in the car with a family friend and other children, a collision had propelled her into the rearview mirror and through the wind-shield. The glass had slashed just above her hairline and caused a "de-gloving injury," the medical term for a scalping. Her scalp had been slipped off like a glove, front to back. One of the other children had been killed, but the girl with whom Donna had just switched places had hardly been injured. Her migraines dated from that injury. On the other hand, her plastic surgeon had done such an expert job that not a sign of the injury showed on her forehead, Donna's dazzling copper-red hair billowing out from her scalp line as though nothing had ever happened. But soon, when Clatterbuck shaves her scalp for surgery, the bright scar of that old wound will stand out in relief.

"Are you more relaxed now?" The nurse is asking. Laurel Moore, the anesthesiologist and a graduate neurointensivist, has just given her a shot to make her drowsy, the first step as they take her down to unconsciousness.

"I feel okay. Yeah, more relaxed," Donna says, the bright red hair poking from beneath the surgical cap. "But my head still —" She makes a ballooning motion with her hands. "And I'm scared. I'm scared." But her voice is so calm, matter-of-fact, that it seems like a clinical observation, perhaps the admission of someone who won't lie to herself.

By coincidence, all Soja's medical attendants are women, gathered above her in that circle of masked faces. "Do you have kids?" from behind a mask.

"Three boys."

"I have a son and daughter," another mask says, eyes laughing. "My son gets a devilish look sometimes, but he is something special. I love my daughter but my son is special."

Another voice comments on how terrifically her fiancé treats his mother. Donna says brightly, "My husband is one of four boys. I'll tell you, his mother wants for nothing."

And somewhere after that the circle fades to black, and Donna exits, as all do under the blanket of deep anesthesia. So different from sleep, when despite a solid night's worth without waking, we come around knowing that time has passed. Donna Soja closes her eyes, and opens them to a different kind of pain in her head, dulled by medication but now the pain of flesh wounds. And a desperate thirst. The cold steel tube in her throat, protruding from her mouth, makes speaking impossible.

It is 7:25 p.m., afternoon stitched directly to evening, and they are unhooking her monitors at the operating table, preparing to slide her onto the gurney for PACU—the Post Anesthesia Care Unit, better known as Recovery. The respiratory therapist is at her side. "Hi, sweetie. You waking up?" Donna struggles, flails at the tubes protruding from her mouth. This is a normal recovery; she will not need the uncomfortable steel intubation tube down her throat. With residents and nurses holding Donna, Moore extubates her in one smooth, briefly painful, sliding motion.

"Cold, cold," Donna croaks. The feeling is common enough coming up from anesthesia that it offers no hint of whether she was in hypothermia or not. She is brought to the Neuro Intensive Care Unit, where she can be closely watched for a few days to make sure she remains stable. They will do what they can to prevent vasospasm, but if that potentially deadly event begins, it probably will not be for nearly a week.

"Drink," Donna says.

Clatterbuck has joined the neurointensivist team in her room. "We can't give you anything to drink tonight, Donna," he says. "You've just had surgery. And it's possible we might need to get you back to the OR. But tomorrow we'll get you a drink."

Laurel Moore checks in on her. "Very, very, very thirsty," Donna tells her.

Turning to the others, Clatterbuck orders medication to help bring sleep through her desperate thirst, and adds, "I'm gonna order a nicotine patch for her. I'll put it on postop orders." And he commits his words to paper. More paper. Everyone in the unit is either writing or carrying a clipboard and pen or pencil, jotting, reading jots. Nurses, techs, doctors all making their marks. Moving fingers write, then write some more, leaving slowly accreting mountains of data like the boulder moraines of glaciers. Nothing gets to residents and fellows quite the way paperwork does, especially at the end of another hard day. Friday is finally over. It is after midnight, Saturday morning. A few yards from where Donna Soja sleeps peacefully, nurse Holli Takahashi holds up a patient chart and says to Chere Chase, who is on hold on the phone, "I hate to say these words to you: summary orders on this patient." More paperwork for Dr. Chase.

"Drive a stake into my heart," Chere says.

S O   E N D S   D O N N A   S O J A ' S first day as a single character in a small play of medical history. She is now a participant in a controlled clinical trial. But what, exactly, does that mean? Begin at the beginning. Scientists may not experiment on people in the same sense they experiment on animals. They may not knowingly cause harm. Even when experimenting on animals, they must follow careful procedures to avoid undue pain and suffering, but they may not in the usual sense "experiment" on people at all, in the sense of trying something to see if it will have the predicted effect.

What this means is that when a new drug or procedure is tried out because it has shown success in animals, the administering physicians must make sure no harm comes to the patient. Whether the procedure works at all—that is, has efficacy—is a separate and less important question in such a Phase I clinical trial. The important question is, Is the experimental procedure *at worst* benign? That answer must be provided to the National Institutes of Health, the usual sponsor of such trials, or to whatever agency is supporting the study. When applying for a Phase I trial grant, the first hurdles to leap are with the hospital's institutional review board, or IRB. The physicians, nurses, and administrators on that board must be shown that the trial will not harm participants.

Success in Phase I might lead to the granting of Phase II funding, and Phase II might be carried out by a growing number of investigators in partnership across the country, or even around the world. It might become a giant, multicenter trial involving hundreds of doctors, thousands of patients, like IHAST2. In addition to Donna Soja and Rita Serianni, dozens of others here have agreed to take part in IHAST2. Eventually, investigators plan to enroll 900 patients worldwide in hopes of answering the question, Does chilling the patient during anesthesia lead to improved outcomes in brain aneurysm surgery? In Phase II, physicians will want to determine efficacy: Does the treatment under study work better than that offered as a standard? Or does it work as well, with fewer side effects? That would be another way of judging it better. Are there side effects? Does the risk of serious side effects wash out potential gain?

In the case of IHAST2, the trial compares two treatments during a particularly risky neurosurgery. But, getting back to the key point, if the patients are randomized, how is this not an experiment on them? It is not an experiment because, regardless of hunches, inclinations, or single case reports, the doctors really do not know which treatment works better. If all goes well, in funding as well as findings, enter Phase III.

Can this thick forest of protections ever be penetrated by error? Can death in the form of a terrible misjudgment slip past so many layers of care? Yes, with shocking ease, as it turns out. Right here at Johns Hopkins Hospital. At Bayview, a young woman named Ellen Roche died less than two months ago, a few days before Mirski boarded the train for grand rounds in New York. She did not die of an error committed at Bayview, but from a drug she took as part of a clinical trial here at Johns Hopkins. She was a healthy volunteer in a study, and she worked in the hospital. She died under the best care available, over a period of agonizing weeks, despite every effort to save her. Her death will resound here soon, threatening hundreds of millions of dollars in research protocols at once.

SATURDAY ROUNDS. The new hospital year is already wearing into a tiring pattern. When Chere Chase gets off call around noon, she plans to nap, then drive straight through to Pittsburgh. Instead, she will oversleep and get to Pittsburgh Sunday, spend the night with her mother, drive on to Cleveland, spend 15 minutes with her boyfriend, turn around and drive back here for Monday rounds. She never misses call, misses few meetings. But what she is missing, hanging like a cloud moving in on her day by day, is a focused research agenda. Half the fellows' time is planned for research under the Johns Hopkins neurointensivist program. That's not saying that the clinical side takes up only 20 hours a week, but that the fellows, as they did as residents in an academic program, must budget time to develop solid agendas of research into important clinical matters on which they can publish in medical journals—initially as second or third authors with attendings or peers, but more and more as lead authors. She and Diana Greene-Chandos have been tireless in the unit, but they have been slow to develop their research.

Further disrupting her schedule, Chase will eventually moonlight to begin paying off medical training debts. She will do physical exams for the Maryland Transit Association in workmen's compensation cases, serving as an intake specialist on Saturday afternoons. Despite her money concerns, she considers herself luckier than many. Because she had spent a year here several years ago getting a health science master's, she was considered a Maryland resident when she entered medical school, so she paid in-state tuition. The class after hers had to go beyond that public health training in order to establish residency. Still, the loans had piled up through four years of med school and four years of postgraduate neurology training at Case Western before she came here. Now, though she was studying as a fellow, the loans had come due. Post-residency training does not qualify for loan deferment. As a fellow, she's earning in the neighborhood of $40,000 a year and helping support her mother as well as herself. Her loans total more than $100,000.

Mike Williams, who is attending on rounds this morning, is feeling weariness as well, for him the annual end-of-July burnout. "I'm exhausted," he says. "The attendings have taken it on ourselves to stay with the new fellows and residents through that first month." Thus the tiredness. But "by staying this week, I've already learned a lot about our two new fellows. It always amazes me. They have different learning styles, different reactions to stress." He says this while standing by Donna Soja's bed, in the corner at the entrance to the unit where the most serious cases tend to spend at least their first hours. He is thinking of Greene-Chandos now, of her most recent crisis.

That patient in crisis was Rita Serianni. Serianni had been recovering well but because the intensivists were concerned about vasospasm, they decided to move her from Bayview, which was still in its first month under their aegis, to the main NICU here. Apparently on the ambulance trip over, Serianni suffered a cerebral herniation, which can be fatal and in any case is an emergency of the first order. *Herniation* refers to a tissue's puffing out through a weakness in surrounding restraint, usually muscle or bone. The typical hernia many people suffer in their abdomens occurs when intestine breaks through such weakness in the overlying abdominal muscle. But the brain swollen from fluid can also herniate, pushing through any of the openings in the surrounding skull. In this case, swelling had caused Serianni's brain to push into the hole at the base of the skull through which the spinal cord rises into the brain stem, called the foramen magnum. But the brain tissue had not, in our commonly used sense of the term, "ruptured." The tissue had not broken; it was being squeezed by pressure. Initially, Rita showed few signs of any problem, and Greene-Chandos was unaware of what had happened, so now she was concerned that she had missed some vital sign, brief though the time lapse was, that would lead to a bad outcome.

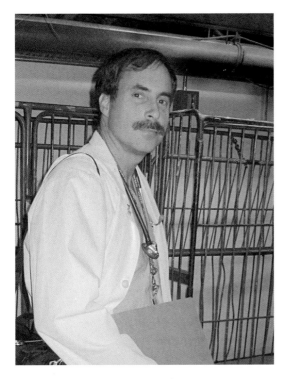

Marek Mirski on the run to Radiology to perform neuroanesthesia. *I wanted to get in the game, to intervene aggressively.*

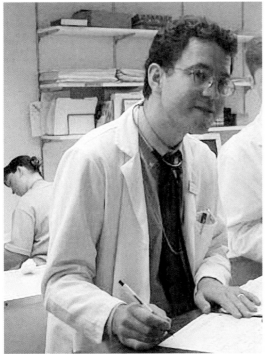

Stephan Mayer engages in the give and take of Columbia rounds. *Our patients are our teachers.... We are doing things so cutting-edge neither we nor anybody else has reams of experience.*

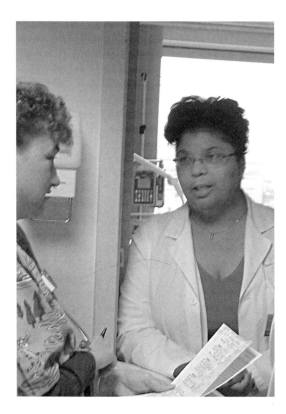

Chere Chase leading rounds at Bayview Medical Center. *There are three medals in the Olympics, her mother always said. But only one of them is gold.*

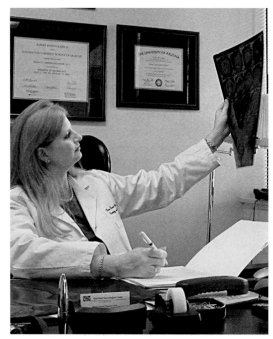

Diana Greene-Chandos studying brain scans in her office. *All I want is to be the best possible doctor.*

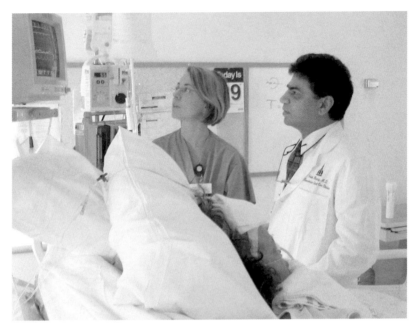

Anish Bhardwaj runs through a patient's "numbers" with nurse Heather Dougherty. *The more we learn, the more patients we can save. Yet so often, you do all you can do and people die.*

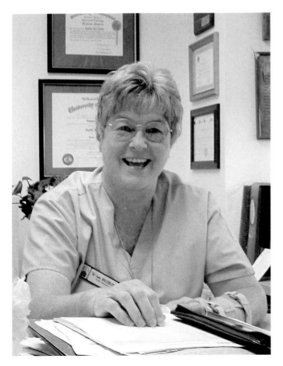

Ski Lower reviews her packed schedule. *There's no nursing crisis here. Our nurses don't leave.*

Jay Lokeman at the home of his sister. *My mother's nicest kid, his brother says. Rippin' and runnin' is about to cut him down.*

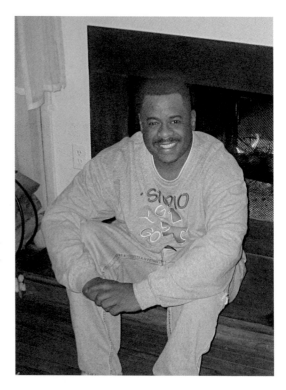

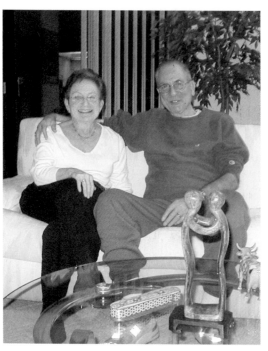

Ellen and Jack Apple during a pleasant evening at home. *An ordinary morning becomes a nightmare drive through the streets of Baltimore.*

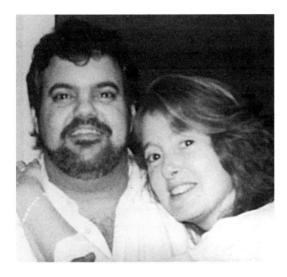

Joe and Gail Beck sharing good times. *How can a solid family be torn by a mosquito dancing on the summer air?*

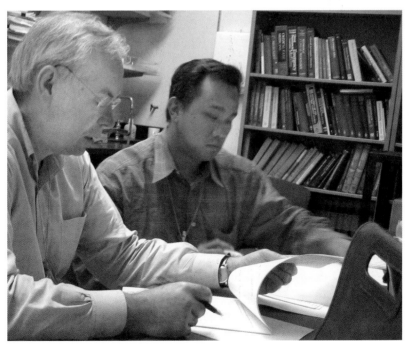

Dan Hanley and Romer Geocadin go over data in the Brain Injury Outcomes lab. *Sometimes when we presume the outcome is fatal, and give up, it becomes fatal.*

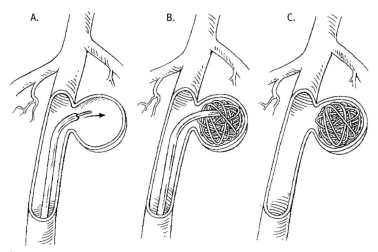

A.   B.   C.

Blocking a killer

A high-tech metal coil is fed from its catheter into the bulb of an aneurysm. Made of "memory metal," the wire automatically balls up to seal off the deadly weakness in the blood vessel.

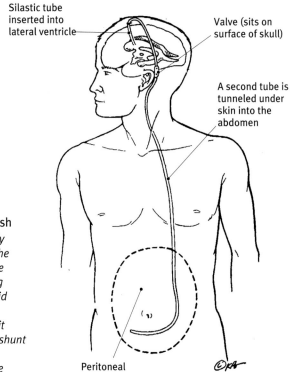

Silastic tube inserted into lateral ventricle

Valve (sits on surface of skull)

A second tube is tunneled under skin into the abdomen

Avoiding the crush

Potentially deadly pressure within the brain can often be eased by draining cerebrospinal fluid from within the ventricles where it forms. This "VP" shunt runs from the ventricles into the peritoneal cavity.

Peritoneal cavity

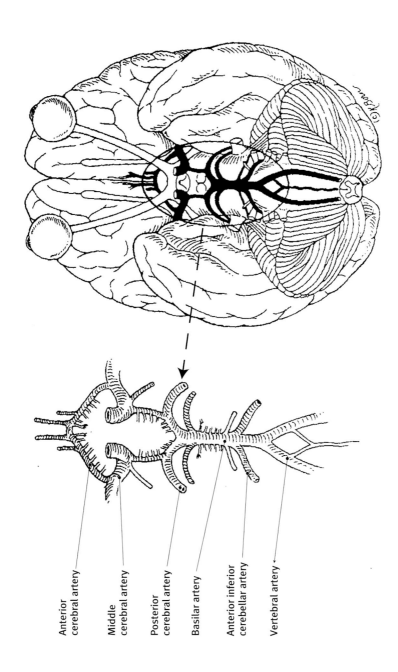

Anterior cerebral artery

Middle cerebral artery

Posterior cerebral artery

Basilar artery

Anterior inferior cerebellar artery

Vertebral artery

Circle of life
The linked arteries of the circle of Willis, lying at the base of the skull, are the most crucial of the brain's blood carriers. If one artery is partially blocked, others in the circle can help restore blood flow.

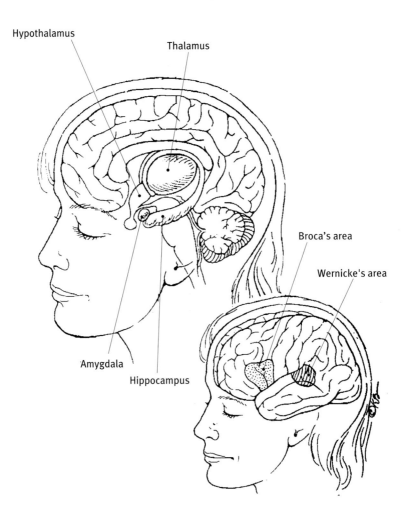

The mind's underground
Critical brain areas in Back From the Brink *are shown upper left and lower right. The larger illustration shows the thalamus and hypothalamus, the major communication crossroads between upper and lower brain. Curved below them is the hippocampus, a critical area for learning and remembering, which terminates in the amygdala. Lower right highlights two vital areas for speech that can be damaged in a stroke. Broca's area controls forming and speaking words. Wernicke's is critical for language comprehension.*

Williams thought not. The problem had been caught as soon as Rita began "posturing," one of the movements associated with moving into coma. "I really don't believe there will be lasting damage from this," Williams said. With brain pressure relieved, "the problem is gone now. Any damage will be from the bilateral strokes last week." Because of the complexity of the aneurysms she suffered, Rita now had lost the blood supply of both frontal anterior cerebral arteries. Would collateral blood flow make up the difference? Quite possibly; and quite possibly not. Williams thought that Serianni would recover, but might lose some brain function. On the more likely side would be losses in "initiation," the ability to make decisions and initiate purposeful action. This could range from the mildest degree, in which she would be no worse off than many otherwise normal people who have the "psychological" failing of indecisiveness, to the most serious, in which she would not be able to string together the self-directed actions needed to get dressed, eat, or take rudimentary care of herself. In that more serious case, for example, she might be able to follow a command to put her shoes on, but could not initiate the action on her own. In other words, the future held a staggering range of possibilities, given her injury, from the mild to the awful, and it would take many months to find out which would emerge as reality.

Phil and the Seriannis' daughters are by Rita's side constantly, talking to her, holding her hand. Often she responds, although the degree of her awareness is unclear.

Serianni is still in the NICU but has been moved down two rooms from where she arrived. Now Donna Soja is in Rita's former bed. A simpler aneurysm but otherwise a remarkably similar case: two women who smoke, one young, one middle-aged, with bleeding aneurysms, occupying the same bed within two days. Do things come in threes? This time they do. With similarities and differences, number three is on the way.

By eight o'clock last night, Carlos Bagley, neurosurgery resident on first call, had already logged in a gunshot wound—a member of the local "knife and gun club"—and traumatic neck injuries to three brothers, who were all riding in the back of a truck, and who all fell off. By the time Bagley saw them they lay in the ER, stretched side by side in identical white collars. But they had escaped major neck or skull injury, so passed from Bagley's purview.

Williams says to Bagley as rounds reach John B____: "Here is another rock in our garden, Carlos. He's chugging along, getting better." But B____ is not going to be a rock this morning. The 72-year-old man is anxious to get up, rolls and swings his legs off the bed and reveals a hospital gown stained with blood—but in smears, not the efflorescence from a wound beneath the gown. His nose is bleeding. "Have you been wiping your nose with your gown, Mr. B____?" Williams says.

"He just did that," nurse Heidi Meyers says. "Ough! I don't put up with blood in my rooms, Mr. B____," she says.

They continue rounding, leaving Meyers to take care of him. "His chest is like the sky this morning," Williams says of another patient. "Scattered clouds but not overcast. Puzzling."

Donna Soja is "superb" today, Williams remarks happily. She is groggy but coming around. Four to nine days from now should tell her recovery story. She either will suffer vasospasm or not; an artery, unpredictable, dangerous, will clamp down for reasons they don't quite underestand, or not. There is strong suspicion, though, that the ever-present villain excitotoxicity is at work in vasospasm. By shortly after 10 a.m., Soja's bed is empty. She has been moved out of intensive care.

AS MORNING ROUNDS BEGAN, a few miles away in north Baltimore the Ray household was stirring. Jennie, 22, home from Vassar and working for a Johns Hopkins unit on a Web site as her summer job, was in the bathroom. Her mother, Nancy Boyd Ray, was in the kitchen, and father, John, was at the table. Nancy heard Jennie groan loudly and ran to the bathroom. In a few minutes the couple had bundled their daughter into their car and were hurrying to Johns Hopkins.

A few hours later, Williams, Chase, residents, and radiology staff are looking over Jennie's scans.

"Jennie Ray, 22. What is that way over there?"

Williams: "That's the pineal gland."

"There? Look at that midline shift!" Not a good sign. The midline is the cleavage between left and right hemispheres of the brain and, as the name implies, the middle is precisely where it should show up at every level of scanning. Any shift indicates brain swelling, either from edema, water, or blood but in any case nothing good.

"Look at all that blood." Indeed, her ventricles contain blood. The lateral horn on her right ventricle, resembling a moose antler in its fullest view, is bright with blood. The hemorrhage will turn out to be caused not by an aneurysm in this case but by an arteriovenous malformation, a congenital disruption in the formation of the lacy artery-vein connections. The neurologists know that such a bleed bathes part of the occipital lobe, where light coming into the eyes is turned into vision, in an area called the calcarine fissure. They will see its effects soon.

Despite the similarity of our genes and their protein products, and the similarity of scans of our brains, there is an amazing diversity that is perfectly normal in the routes arteries and veins take when forming during fetal development and in the explosion of growth afterward. The brain's neurons follow signals as they send their axonal projections sliding along to often-distant targets, billions at a time, tugged by their outward-growing growth cones that for all the world give the appearance that the axon is being towed by an amoeba. Neurons themselves migrate throughout the embryo's cortex. Neuroscientists are still unsure of the mechanisms at work.

Some of the new cells become "hearing" neurons, others "seeing," and still others will be involved in touch or making decisions about what motion to carry out next. Do they start out as subtly different cells, already destined for those very different roles? Or are they identical neurons, whose function becomes determined solely by where they wind up? The latter appears to be the case, strange as that seems, for it leads to a paradox. If the hearing cortex contains neurons identical to those in the visual system, in what sense does it "hear"? And similarly for the billions of visual system neurons, at what level do they "see"? In other words, at what level of circuitry do the enormous qualitative differences in sensory experience emerge?

Arteries are not programmed to end up in specific locations, either. Branches sprout and head off in response to a demand for blood. Look at the scans of six normal people and you will see amazing variation in the branch points and twists of even the largest arteries, all of which may function perfectly. And then there are the nonnormal ways that they can form. The arteriovenous malformation, or AVM, is common among these abnormalities. As any X ray shows, a major artery branches like tumbleweed, each branch point leading to finer offshoots until the vascular system reaches the near-microscopic level. There, in the brain, astrocytes wrap their footlike projections tightly around the smallest arterial capillaries, forming the blood-brain barrier. On the other side of the oxygen delivery system, the venous drainage, the largest of the veins is fed by ever dwindling streams of smaller veins, down to filaments the size of the smallest arteries. Here capillary meets capillary, outgoing complementing incoming. These smallest veins pick up blood drained of its oxygen, which had been delivered to cells by the smallest arteries. Why is that important? Because at that cellular level, the arterial pressure is lowest, and it is matched to what the veins can stand. Fluctuations in blood pressure caused by excitement or physical activity are spread through the whole system of millions of tiny capillaries. If you stand suddenly, the pressure jolt is finely distributed and absorbed. In the misformed structure called an AVM, the smaller tributaries do not form correctly, and sometimes do not form at all. Sizeable arteries link to sizable veins. With nothing to absorb sudden changes in blood pressure, sooner or later, just as at the weak point in an aneurysm, the juncture pops. That's what had happened to Jennie Ray this morning.

Yet lying in bed in the NICU, she alternately seems okay, then fades to sleepiness, then comes back again. That's the appearance. "Where do you go to school?" Williams asks her. "Sarah Lawrence," she says, incorrectly. "What are you majoring in?" "English," she says correctly. Her voice is clear; she simply seems distracted by something.

"On a scale of one to ten, how much does your head hurt?"

"Seven and a half," she says smartly. In and out.

But by noon, she is thrashing in pain, holding her head, kicking her legs out. Williams says, "If we do anything today, it'll be a catheter, to drain her vents," because the ventricles are being pressurized with blood, and they need to be drained to prevent pressure from building in the surrounding brain.

"Do you know what happened to you?" Williams says.

"I'm in the living room, that's all. And I have a terrrible headache."

"You're in Johns Hopkins Hospital."

No response. Then she is annoyed, peevish at being disturbed. "I can't see because your hand is over my eyes." But Williams is feet away from her, and her eyes are open, staring.

"Do you wear any [dental] braces?"

"Not anymore." Clear as a bell. "I wear a retainer at night."

"We need to get Jennie intubated fast, to protect her airway," Williams says. "Then we'll worry about the catheter."

An hour later, behind the door that still has Donna Soja's name on it, Jennie is vomiting and writhing. An anesthesiologist sweeps in, intubation kit in hand. "What has she had?" "Twenty-five of fentanyl," the heavyweight painkiller used in anesthesia. Fentanyl is a frequently prescribed painkiller in both OR and ICU, and in the right hands is a gift of medical science. Clumsily used, it can be deadly, as the Russians proved when they used it to knock out terrorists holding hostages in Moscow and killed scores of the hostages.

Once intubation is completed, Williams says to the resident, "Why don't you take Jennie downstairs" for brain scans. "I'll watch things up here. You"—to Chere—"go home. Drive carefully. Sleep if you need to." She leaves for what she intends to be a quick nap. Williams orders out for pizza for the crew. Most Saturdays are quiet. "Two or three Saturdays a year it's like this," he says. "I just ask one of the nurses to order us food. Gotta eat."

Jennie's mother, Nancy, sits alone in her room, maternal concerns translated into a determined confidence, a resolute optimism of outcome. She and her husband, John, brought Jennie here themselves at the suggestion of their family doctor. Had they called an ambulance, it would have taken her to whichever hospital was on its rotation list for neurological emergencies, a system used in most cities to prevent single hospitals from drawing all the trauma cases. But John and Nancy had wanted her here. "Then take her to the Johns Hopkins ER yourselves," the doctor had advised.

"She is a terrifically active student at Vassar," Nancy Boyd says. "She's going to be a senior in the fall. She's in the Madrigal Singers. She's just as bright and active as can be." Perhaps by conjuring these truths and willing them, they will remain so in the future.

Williams explains that Rafael Tamargo, the vascular neurosurgeon, will be in soon to insert the catheter that, if all goes well, will keep the pressure in Jennie's head steady. Williams says, "Unlike an aneurysm, the likelihood of an AVM rebleeding on the first day is fairly small—about 5 percent—so there's no need to do something acutely. There's no need for emergency surgery, coiling or anything." He is more concerned about the possibility of hydrocephalus, and that is his own area of expertise. A sudden rise in blood pressure in the brain, swelling in the brain or ventricles, could disrupt the brain stem controls for breathing. So Jennie will be kept intubated and prepared for a ventilator until they are sure she is out of danger. "I don't like the way she falls asleep in midsentence," he says. "She's not out of the woods yet."

"Jennie is going to write a creative work for her senior thesis," Nancy Boyd says determinedly. "Some of the better students in English can elect to do that, but it will mean a very busy year."

Back from being scanned, Jennie Ray has been found to have 2.5 cc's of blood in the lateral horns of her ventricles, a good-size hemorrhage, but it is no longer bleeding, so there is an excellent chance for complete recovery.

Just after 7 p.m., Rafael Tamargo and his resident arrive at Jennie's side, gowned for surgery. Everyone else leaves as they roll an instrument table across her bed, then scrub in, in order to place the intraventricular catheter drain right here at bedside. Williams and Tamargo go over the scans together: there is shrinkage of the intraventricular spaces, so the brain is being squeezed. Tamargo rattles off the medications he'll be using, to eliminate pain and block any memory she might ordinarily have of the procedure, since she is not being put into the near-coma of general anesthesia. Using a hand drill, the resident bores a small hole into the skull bone. The drill, with its crank wheel, looks identical to those sold at hardware stores and is a reminder that, at the end of all the high technology, neurosurgery and the intensive care of the brain are still mostly about hand tools and skilled hands. Then the resident pushes the thin catheter carefully into the skull opening, slipping it between the meninges but seeing no fluid welling up at him. "We're not in," he says. He and Tamargo exchange words softly until, on the third try, "Got it." Spinal fluid wells powerfully into the catheter. This fluid, as expected, is bloody.

They can tell the pressure is high, so, "Good call" on inserting the catheter, Tamargo says to Williams.

Down the hall, Donna Soja is awake and alert just 24 hours after surgery. She is remembering the degloving accident when she was 10, how luckily the house right behind the crash site was home to a young woman on vacation from nursing school, who helped her and the others out of the glass-strewn car and onto her patio, to await the ambulances. John Soja looks more tired than she. He had driven two hours to get home to Dover after a long yesterday, caught a few hours sleep, then driven two hours back today. He would go home to be with the kids tonight.

In the next room, Rita Serianni is frowning, breathing hard. "I'll suction you," the nurse says gently, and does so. In the hall a nurse walks by wearing a T-shirt that reads, JOHNS HOPKINS NEUROSCIENCES . . . OUTWIT, OUTLAST. Harder than it sounds.

In George R____'s room, Williams and the neurosurgery resident talk over problems with R____'s family, of a frequent sort. A son and daughter are at odds with a second son over their father's treatment and prognosis, and the prognosis is not good. The latter son has not arrived at the hospital until a few days ago, and he is angry at the dark forecast, angry that not enough is being done. It is common—often after weeks of a family's watching a loved one meteorically rise and fall only to begin a final downward spiral—for a long-absent member to show up and want to "take it from the top," to begin the whole course of treatment as though the crisis had just begun. It is so common that the latecomer is referred to in hospital parlance as "the child from the other coast."

A few doors away, Ardelia Lokeman talks with her children, who are all gathered round. Jay is resting before them but gaining strength day by day. Son Vernon, she recalls, chiding him kiddingly, was born right near here in Halsted, weighing in at 9 pounds 3 ounces after keeping her in labor for 24 hours. Daughter Cathy also was born in Halsted, but Jay was delivered at Lutheran Hospital. Son Joey, who got here a little later than the rest, had to fly in from The Hague, where he had been attending a jazz festival. The sound at their backs is not usual for a hospital, let alone a Neurointensive Care Unit—hammering, coming from where the new NICU is under construction. But it's intermittent on this Saturday night, as though left behind to remind of the wholesale crashing and machine gun fire of pneumatic tools of the weekdays.

Exiting Jay Lokeman's room, a month ago you would turn left and head out to the family waiting room. Now that door is blocked with a row of lockers, the din of reconstruction going on right beyond. A sign posted on the lockers features a cartoon Leaning Tower of Pisa with a crane straightening it. PARDON OUR PROGRESS, it says.

"That sign cost $3.5 million," quips one of the residents.

CHAPTER 9

Drive, Drive, Drive

WHAT DRIVES the inhabitants of the world collectively called neuro intensive? Start with drive at its most literal, muscle power, as in Drive for the goal. Responding to the catastrophes that bring patients to the brink of death, where only physical intervention has a prayer of keeping them alive, is the first order of the hospital day, and the need for that physical action unites the neurointensivists of this story more than any other single quality.

Here it is, literal as it gets. Tuesday rounds so far have proceeded unremarkably, Romer Geocadin leading as attending this week. But something about the next case grabs everyone's close attention. You could watch it being discussed without sound and see it is out of the ordinary, from each person's body language. These are doctors who never lose their cool or raise their voices, who try never to let anger or upsetment edge into their talk—at least not in the NICU. Their body language is normally muted as well. But now, as the nurse or neurology resident recites or reads from a chart, all heads turn, first to the speaker, then toward the darkened room. Inside is Josefa M____.

In a flophouse not far from here on Broadway, in the middle of last night, a man who lived there heard loud moaning. It went on and on. Finally looking in, he saw a woman naked on the bed, covered in blood. One eye was swollen shut and her belly was swollen with the last weeks of pregnancy. Nurse Heidi Meyers related what was passed along from the emergency room, which came largely from the ambulance crew that brought her in. EMTs were called to the rooming house. They found Josefa lying there, a teddy bear next to her; blood stained the sheets and spotted the walls and ceiling. The police were already there. Josefa's husband had returned sometime after the EMTs left with her, and he had been arrested.

In emergency surgery a few hours ago, the trauma surgeon had removed a brain clot. Josefa was found to be in labor, one centimenter dilated and contracting. The fetus was estimated at 37 to 38 weeks based on size, nearly full term. By the end of her neurosurgery, she was three centimeters dilated, so her surgeon made a judgment call for a C-section, and that was performed. She had delivered an apparently healthy baby boy.

"So what do we know?" Geocadin asks, to strip the sad drama to its neurointensive essentials. "We don't really know anything." And he begins reading off his observations, rapid-fire: "Blown left pupil, diagonally ovoid. Preferential gaze to the right? Possibly." A brain hemorrhage on the left, given its location on the scans they now huddle around, is dangerous even if not deadly. The clot removed was in or near speech areas. "She could have language problems, aphasia," he says. Aphasia is the term for any loss of language ability, either in speaking or comprehending. Language, as we've seen, is mapped onto fairly well defined regions of the brain, usually in the left hemisphere. Patients' loss of particular language skills became the first major evidence, as far back as the nineteenth century, that the brain was in fact a global federation of largely localized functions. That known, the visible damage to Josefa's brain suggests functional loss later, but only suggests. No two brains have precisely the same boundaries for language or most other functions.

Now comes the careful discussion of what to do for the young woman, matching all the particulars of her case against the common dangers they are trained to tackle. Whether you are recovering from a craniotomy for tumor and membranes have been cut to expose brain tissue to air, or you've had a hemorrhage and the brain was exposed to blood, or even if you've suffered the kind of ischemic stroke that might leave no observable effects for days—these are just different roads to the same dangerous place. The NICU team must work to reduce brain swelling. Until they gain control over swelling, contrary to what was standard practice a few years ago, they generally must not reduce blood pressure—yet reducing blood pressure would seem intuitive if a blood vessel has burst. If blood pressure were reduced now, the high intracerebral pressure of the swelling could choke healthy arteries, and that in turn could kill even more brain. The doctors must also look for the emergence of excitatory neurotransmitters such as glutamate into the spaces between brain cells, where they and their breakdown chemicals and other by-products of a cell's violent death can poison through excitotoxicity.

Finally, for the neurointensivists as case managers, are there signs that any other organs are failing? Most commonly and dangerously, that would be lungs or kidneys. In this closed Neuro ICU, until they call in a specialist consultant, the patient is all theirs. That is the feature that varies the most widely among the neurointensivist programs throughout the country, but the one on which Mirski, like Hanley before him, is most adamant. Unless one physician is in charge of the whole patient, Mirski says, "You have a group of chefs, each with their own recipe and not knowing what effect it has on the others."

As always, there is the particular insult or infection that must be attacked in this case; then there are the common consequences that follow in the badly injured brain, which often take priority because they are constant killers or cripplers. You can spend an entire summer and hear of one case of encephalitis, but you cannot pass a morning without hearing of the major dangers that ensue in virtually every critical-care patient. Blood flow, brain pressure, cytotoxicity. Lungs. Kidneys. The short list.

They move on, pushing the cart between them carrying patient records and their own notes, a crew as international as you will see in any hospital, and hospital crews are all international. Western medicine is a lodestone worldwide, drawing the best and brightest from every continent. And mixed among the foreign medical school graduates, of course, is the multi-everything mix of American demographics.

Next morning, as the team moves to her bed, they see a form no different from yesterday's. _"Josefa! Dame su mano, Josefa . . . Abierta mi mano."_ _Nada._ But the monitors sweep and measure, the nurses watched frequently all night, the resident examined her before rounds this morning, and, merging that data with all their observations, they find reason for optimism. Though subtle, all the signs say Josefa M____ is improving. Her healthy baby boy is in the neonatal ward. The husband who beat her bloody had been selling her for sex in return for drugs. He is in jail. Over the next few days, she rises steadily out of coma into a state of unaware wakefulness and sleep, not knowing who or where she is yet, but able to respond, day by day a bit more. Then another few days and she will be herself again, whoever that may be. The social worker following her case comes in to see her often, and soon Josefa is released to move in with relatives in New York City, the worker reports. And then, in the curt language of medical demographics, Josefa and her baby are lost to follow-up.

IN THE HALL OF MIRRORS of the brain, nothing stays literal for long. Drive is just the word for the obsessions that set people in motion when they're alone as well as physically engaged. There is the drive called ambition, ego-drive. The drive to succeed is a rich part of the mix at any of the world's top academic institutions. And there is the drive to see what cannot be seen, maybe among the most powerful of all motivators of pure research—to satisfy a craving to discover.

At the conclusion of rounds, Geocadin hurries off to meet with Dan Hanley, who is mentoring the major funded project for which Geocadin is principal investigator—the investigation into cardiac arrest deaths and recoveries. He heads toward the warren of offices and research space where Hanley is carving out a laboratory as head of the Division of Brain Injury Outcomes. In this routine, scheduled meeting, they will go over the latest data for the study that is shaping Geocadin's research, and that research will power his early years as an assistant professor, a scientist-clinician.

Of medium height and athletically built, Geocadin has the dark skin and almond eyes of his native Philippines. He is quick to smile in the NICU and to laugh uproariously in less severe settings. His intensity shows in the enthusiasm and passion with which he discusses this or any project, as Hanley's shows in the spacing between words and the quiet emphasis on them. Romer and his wife, Effie, came to like Baltimore slowly. They missed New York City. Training as a neurology resident at

New York University, his duty hours were spent in the trauma and emergency hot spot of Bellevue Medical Center. Action was constant. The riches of New York were at hand. Their apartment was within blocks of Lincoln Center, where they could take in plays, the opera, symphonies.

But then, Geocadin's roots were far from there, too. Born and raised on the large island of Negros Occidental, in the center of the Philippine archipelago but a long way from Manila, he was one of four children, his father a lawyer in the port city of Bacolod. Not every high achiever has a formative experience. But for Romer there was such an experience, though not a happy one.

When his younger sister was 7 years old, she fell ill with vomiting and dizzy spells. Doctors first said the problem was just in her eyes and would go away. She seemed to recover, then got sick again. Then she began having trouble walking. Finally, his parents took her to the nearest island that had a neurologist. The diagnosis was terrifying: she had a brain tumor. But even the neurologist couldn't tell them more than that, because he had no access to a scanner. The one CT scanner in the entire Philippines was in Manila, a 90-minute flight. So the Geocadins all set off for the capital, where they were told an operation was his sister's best chance, and that was only 50-50. Her struggle had been long and painful. With some misgivings, the Geocadins decided to have the operation. The girl died months later. The whole family was devastated, the kind of experience that turns many away from modern fixes, even leaves them embittered. But Romer remembered his father saying in frustration, "Why don't we have people to solve these problems?" He decided that would be him.

He attended the University of the East in Manila, then went to Ramon Magsaysay Medical School. There the dean, Harvard-trained neurologist Joven Cuanang, so inspired Romer's entire class that nearly a dozen of his peers went into neurology. After NYU-Bellevue, he completed his neurointensivist fellowship here at Johns Hopkins in 1999. He and his friend Ricardo Carhuapoma were among the last Hanley trainees, and when Ricardo set off for Columbia, Romer became an attending physician and assistant professor at this most academic of academic medical centers.

Now, between his other duties, Geocadin followed along as a member of the Brain Attack team, the others all stroke specialists, as they hit the ER and ICU, always ready to be paged for a cardiac arrest, the focus of his research. The project takes him from the emergency room in the basement at the north end of the mammoth Hopkins complex up to the seventh floor NICU facing east toward the bay, to laboratory space opposite Hanley's office in an old corner of the Jefferson building, facing west along Broadway. An appropriate expanse, because the project is potentially that far-reaching, and it won Geocadin one of just two prestigious American Academy of Neurology fellowships awarded last year. In some ways, the project also takes him to the farthest remove from the laboratory where he, like Mirski and Bhardwaj, closes in on ever-smaller bits of biological terrain.

Under the intraoperative microscope of neurosurgery, the human brain looms as a giant pink planet, more twisted and rilled with ridges and valleys than the moon, in solidity somewhere between that pale, cold rock and the boiling sun. In its living state, the brain has been described by those who have touched underneath the skin of its meninges as a viscous gel and as having the consistency of cooked oatmeal. Yet it is a thing, the human mind made manifest. Lose the wrong parts of it to tumor, infection, or trauma and that will be perfectly clear to those who knew you when.

More powerful microscopes can parse the brain into cells, the cells into giant worlds of their own, trafficking in nutrients, water, a few vitamins and minerals and shipping out communications in measurable pulses of electrochemistry. The "microscopes" of chemical analysis can spy on the activities of genes too small for the world of light that seeing requires. That journey down is one direction brain science takes, the direction of Mirski's basic research into the internal signaling processes of guinea pig brains as he looked for human analogs.

But you can also start with the whole person as one unit, then draw back as though you were rising above Earth and watch the field of vision expand from one person to a dozen, then a hundred, and so forth. You can keep going as epidemiologists do, until individuals vanish like pixels on a computer screen, blending into whorls and patterns of behavior. Then you can ask questions like this: Why do some people recover from cardiac arrest, like that suffered by Michael Sanders, with no aftereffects, while others make it to the emergency room as fast but make no comeback?

The basics are simple. Each year, 1 million people suffer cardiac arrest, usually idiopathic—of no known cause, unlike Sanders's, which turned out to have been caused by an aneurysmal bleed. But for now cause is beside the point, because virtually all cardiac arrest victims are dead on arrival at the emergency room. Humans cannot tolerate more than a few minutes without oxygen before massive cerebral infarction begins. The brain accounts for only about 2 percent of the average person's body weight, but uses 25 percent of all the oxygen breathed for its never-interrupted daily communications among a hundred billion neurons.

So it is interesting that some patients do make it into and past the ER. Why? More interestingly, of those patients who make it, some recover completely and resume their lives. Why them? Most of those who do make it to the emergency room either never emerge from coma or, worse, linger in the persistent vegetative state that can go on for years. What distinguishes them from those who recover?

It appeared that you could wash out differences in age, gender, and other demographic and lifestyle influences—none seemed to predict good or bad outcome. And then you were left with a mystery: Why does this patient live and that one die?

A fundamental requirement of the scientific method is that you pause before big questions and break them down into operational ones, simpler questions with measurable answers. Whatever the causal machinery behind the patients' different outcomes, would there be something visible on the EEGs of the cardiac arrest patients who survived that did not show up on the EEGs of those who died or remained comatose? Something that might even be a marker for good odds?

It was interesting that some few people with cardiac arrest lived to tell about it—not their memories of the event, which are universally wiped out, but the feat itself. But it was potentially life-saving on a large scale if, by EEG, for example, you could find those patients with the best chance of survival and save them. Instead of, as now at so many hospitals, writing them all off because of the dismal odds.

Geocadin and Hanley sit at a long laboratory bench across from Hanley's office, looseleaf binders containing drafts, notes, graphs pertaining to Geocadin's work spread out between them. What's new?

Geocadin points to findings from other studies, highlighting a direction those investigators did not take, a direction he thinks might prove interesting. Hanley counters with a few citations, publications that might touch on this line of inquiry. Moving on: here in this other data Geocadin thinks there might be something very interesting, or maybe it's just a blip of no consequence; something to look into. There will be this deadline to think about, that conference coming up if results are in. Today's might be the routine encounter between Hanley and Geocadin that, a year hence, is seen as providing the seed of the big breakthrough. More likely nothing of much consequence will come of it. But the accretion of all these moments, observations, and measurements adds up to science as daily life, against which the dramas upstairs stand in such sharp relief. And Geocadin is always excited to talk about his research, eager to explore trajectories that the brief lines of his graphs might soon be taking.

His pilot study lies at the beginning of the labyrinthine process aimed at breaking the causal chains that lead patients to the NICU. Can Geocadin identify a group of cardiac arrest victims likely to benefit from aggressive treatment? If so, his pilot study might be expanded from the number of patients enrolled here, or it might include patients at a few more medical centers, like Robert Fisher's trials of Mirski's thalamic implant. And all that is still very much the opening round in the clinical trial process. Farther along the road to accepted clinical practice are the large, multicenter trials like one in which Hanley himself was now engaged.

M A R E K M I R S K I , driving home a point, jumps the scale from macro to micro on the whiteboard at the front of the meeting room in the NICU, now making a cartoonish cell puff up with the water of edema, now sketching the outcome percentages across the vast realm of patients. Often, we begin pulling together diverse lines of thought as though absently, all the while setting course determinedly, building a case. The drive: to resolve a contradiction, an anomaly, a blur of dangerous uncertainty. Idiopathic means of no known cause. Nothing really happens without cause—at least, that's the faith of rationalists.

Anish Bhardwaj, sitting next to where Mirski stands, is investigating aquaporins in the laboratory. These are the channels that carry water into and out of the brain cell. Except in such cartoons as those on the board, these channels are far too small to be seen even in a neuron drawn the size of a hand. But a cartoon is a visual metaphor, so Mirski's aquaporins are like pipes through the membrane, which itself would be as gossamer-thin as the aquaporin channels through it. Water passes through membranes in the process called osmosis. You can give the water a push out into the blood by boosting blood salt—making the blood "hyper" "osmolar."

"Using hyperosmolar solutions is an area where, basically, this unit has produced the world literature—at least for neuro," Mirski says, repeating for emphasis, "Most of the literature has come out of this unit." Presto, out come the ever-present research papers for inspection, for copying should any of the articles match the attendees' own research interests.

We are pumping salt water into the brain again, but Mirski is going somewhere new this time.

"What can happen if we've got somebody on hypertonic saline" to reduce edema, "and suddenly you give them a big dose of normal fluid?" The question comes at the tail of a long, tortuous path on the board tracing the brain cell's controls as they battle to maintain the cell's size and at the same time keep sodium out. "What can happen?"

A resident: "You can get rebound."

"Right! Excellent. The neurons have adapted a bit to the salt, they're expecting it to be out there trying to pull out their water, so they're countering the salt—but suddenly the salt is not there. They're trying to keep their size up, so now they'll really start filling up with water. The upshot is that if you abruptly stop presenting salt to those cells, you can very quickly get edema as bad or worse than before."

He relates a near-disaster in the unit a few years earlier. "A family member brought one of our patients a two-liter bottle of Diet Coke, which he thirstily drank." Two hours later the patient suffered a brain herniation. "Fortunately we got to him in time, and everything came out well."

As Mirski looks at Greene-Chandos, she is already nodding.

"We had a patient coming over from Bayview," Mirski says of Rita Serianni. "Could that have been the problem?"

"Part of it," she says. "Yes." Serianni was not kept on the high intravenous salt water once she left the Bayview ICU for the ambulance trip to Johns Hopkins, which may have been why she was herniating when she got to Greene-Chandos. Apparently, as Williams had believed, the effects were only temporary. She appeared to have recovered from that problem completely. Nevertheless, what had been a potentially life-threatening crisis now had a cause, and a lesson to be tucked away.

A voice from behind: "Sorry I'm late." Chere Chase has arrived from Pittsburgh in time to take over call from Greene-Chandos. Soon their month of resident's call will be over. There will be more time for research, of just the sort that makes its way into the papers Mirski and Bhardwaj regularly pass around, the sort that drives Johns Hopkins and its brethren.

That drive, when the match is just right, makes a confluence with the investigator's drive to see things that cannot be seen, to resolve contradictions. The research drive is meant to form a feedback loop toward a good end, breeding synergy. Medical calamities, illnesses, the wear of normal living drive the doctor to do research; research finds answers and brings in the funds that, far more than patient-care dollars, keep the institution going.

Yet the match between lab experiment or trial protocol and the "real world" of the unit is anything but smooth. Out here, try as we may, things just aren't well controlled. Mirski once said, "How can you demonstrate that any treatment in the clinical world is better than another?" And he shook his head in response. "In the lab you can control everything. That's why animal models are so important. One of the troubles is, they're animal models. There are physiological differences, some of which we don't understand, that make it difficult or impossible to translate what we've found in the bench world into the clinical world."

For Mirski, the greatest neuroscience example of the difficulty in translating bench research into bedside care can be found in the treatment of
stroke, a topic so much at the fore here in recent days..

"There have been 25 to 50 clinical stroke trials of major magnitude in
the United States—all large, multicenter clinical trials evaluating medications or interventions that had proven themselves in the laboratory in
animal models," Mirski said, "and some of those experiments suggested
a tremendous efficacy." All had proven negative in humans.

Part of this is the difference in physiology. We are all genetically related. The many genes that encode the blueprints for an eye, after all, have
more similarities than differences for any creatures with eyes. But the genetic distance to even our nearest "relatives" is astronomical compared
with the differences among any human beings.

There's also the problem of isolating one disease or one injury as the
major cause of a patient's decline. "Nobody comes into the hospital with
one illness," Mirski said. "You come in with a stroke, but the stroke came
from something—hypertension, diabetes, atrial fibrillation, a number of
other co-morbidities. It's impossible to get a population of patients that are
in any way identical."

Ideally, as a scientist, you would like to have thousands of patients
who were, quite literally, clones. Same age. Same jobs. Same everything,
except for one factor. Say, some smoke cigarettes and some do not. You
learn that not one of the clones who survive cardiac arrest ever smoked.
Or perhaps some survivors had smoked but quit at least ten years ago.
Meanwhile, nearly all those who never drew another breath after cardiac
arrest were smokers. Looking over a field of dots, each representing a patient, that numbered in the thousands—millions would be better—the
answers were always the same. Here would be black and white, approaching
truth to within the tiniest of error bars. That would be great science, but

you would never find such ideal circumstances in the real world. In fact, this is precisely the kind of controlled science researchers attempt to carry out in the laboratory, with animals that indeed might soon be clones and even now are bred for genetic constancy and specific traits. But using them, results are black and white only for guinea pigs, or nude mice—or even chimpanzees, genetically the closest to humans of any living thing, but most certainly not human.

Often the whole point of a clinical trial is to take results that are iron-clad in lab animals and extend them to humans. In Phase I of a clinical trial, all you need to be sure of is that the treatment you proffer does no harm to patients. *Primum non nocere.* First, do no harm. Once you prove your protocol does no harm to any and appears to help some, you can move on through the maze.

If you're using rats as an animal model, you can use rats from the same litter to control for genetic differences. By contrast, if ten laboratory rats could tell you all you needed to know of a problem's cause, Mirski says, it would take a thousand patients to comparably "wash out the variables" to get at a similar problem among humans. And nowhere is the task more difficult than in critical care. A sizable percentage of patients here will die, "and they may not die because of what you're trying to treat with the medicine—but of pneumonia, for example."

TO GET JENNIE RAY DOWNSTAIRS for the angiogram that will show blood flowing through all her brain's arteries and reveal details of her hemorrhage and AVM requires a staff-depleting team from the NICU. One resident, two nurses, and a respiratory therapist line up on either side of Jennie's gurney, rolling it between them, one pushing her wheeled IV pole, another steadying the tubes and wires over the gurney. Down into the basement, which looks like a Disneyland "imagineering" trip to the wrong side of Baltimore. Underground grunge. Gray walls and floors, crates stacked on pallets, dented barrels. The working bowels of the hospital with its industrial laundry room, what looks like a machine shop. Everything but the crash of foundry noise. Not a sound except the rattling of the gurney and footsteps down the long corridor to Radiology. Jennie will get an angiogram with contrast, meaning that radiologist Kieran Murphy will inject a dye that will show up sharply in the images, enabling the neurosurgeon on call to estimate how bad her hemorrhage is and where it lies in relation to the newly found AVM.

To the neurologists here, as noted earlier, none of this beats the neurological exam for revealing the state of a patient's brain. But there's a hitch to conducting that exam in the NICU, for it requires that patients be extubated and not be on medications that would interfere with their level of consciousness.

Murphy, the director of interventional neuroradiology, narrates what he sees as he threads the catheter slowly up through the diminishing arteries into the region of Jennie's AVM. He has the lilting brogue of his native Dublin, where he graduated from medical school; he followed up with residencies and fellowships at Albany Medical Center, the University of Michigan, the University of Geneva, Switzerland. What he is seeing now was fine-tuned at each stop of his training. He is in a subspecialty only metaphorically at the cutting edge of physical interventions into the brain—because these interventions uniquely avoid cutting through the skull and into the brain.

A generation ago, aneurysms that led to hemorrhagic stroke were almost invariably fatal, or so destructive that death often would have been a kindness. The next generation of neurosurgeons, aided by the intraoperative microscope, brought ever-growing numbers of patients to good recoveries. But a host of complications still accompanies brain surgery, and perhaps will for the foreseeable future. For neurosurgeons to clip the neck of an aneurysm, they must retract the brain from its resting place on the shelf of the skull, at what risk is not clear. Everything surrounding the craniotomy poses additional risks, from the deep anesthesia to exposure to air of brain tissue that until that moment had been shielded from infection by its three-layered membrane covering.

Like many aneurysms, AVMs sometimes must be surgically removed; that is, the small region where the capillaries did not form is removed; the neighboring normal vessels gradually pick up the load, and everything returns to normal. Or, if possible, like some aneurysms, AVMs can be coiled. The neurosurgeon or radiologist doing the work watches progress on the TV monitor, showing real-time angiography, as now. There on the monitor the catheter feeds up from the femoral artery in the thigh, through the ghostly carotid artery in the neck, the catheter carrying a thin, high-tech wire at its tip. When the site is reached, the wire is released and automatically balls up, like spaghetti on an invisible fork, and blocks the AVM. Finally, if small enough, the AVM sometimes can be zapped with X rays and sealed off. All the intended outcomes are the same, with normal artery-capillary-vein combinations taking up the slack of the missing branch, oxygenating and feeding the brain.

The introduction of coiling potentially changed all the co-morbidity risks for both problems. Patients can go home in days instead of the weeks required after craniotomy. But which works better in the long term over a wide range of different aneurysms, coiling or clipping? That was the inspiration for the European research protocol in which Murphy is now engaged. In Europe, coiling has long been favored over neurosurgery for amenable aneurysms, and the huge, multicenter European trial that has been under way for several years is now drawing into its final, conclusive phase. Murphy is the only U.S.

investigator in this trial, Johns Hopkins the only participating U.S. medical center.

But Murphy's role today is simply to get detailed pictures to add to those done when Jennie was admitted. Eventually, they will help neurosurgeon Rafael Tamargo decide what course of treatment will be best for her.

Mirski spends much time with Murphy, discussing the radiologist's vision of treatments just over the horizon, because for one day post-procedure, at least, Murphy's coiling patients will be in Mirski's NICU. In addition to the expected increase in neurosurgery patients once the NICU was expanded, the unit would see a boom from those passing through Interventional Neuroradiology. The unit, already stretched thin, will have to meet those demands.

As Murphy works today, members of the team peel off to answer pages or head back upstairs, some wending their way back to the Neuro ICU. This whole round-trip has been in Mirski's sights for a long time. In the new unit he envisioned, staffing would be pressed to the limit. There had to be a better way to protect patients too sick to hand over to the hospital's transport aides, a way that would not consume so much staff time.

Enter the Purple People—as in, people wearing purple scrubs instead of the hospital's usual pale green. They are mostly former staff nurses in need of regular hours, or of moving off the fast track, or who want to work only part-time. They had been part of Johns Hopkins for several years, but soon they would become a key part of solving Mirski's puzzle, and their distinctive uniforms would be seen increasingly in the unit as their wearers pushed gurneys and allowed the NICU staff to stay in place.

T H E   M O R N I N G   S U N   slides across the floor, a beaching breaker. There they go again, the white coats, the pushcart table with the charts, down to Jennie's room. Diana Greene-Chandos has been on resident's call overnight, and here is what she has observed on each rounding: *Jennie is sicker than she knows.*

"Good morning," Greene-Chandos says to Jennie, repeating the phrase precisely on each visit. "My name is Dr. Greene, and I'll be looking after you today. How are you feeling?"

"Nice to meet you, Dr. Greene," Jennie replies every time, in some variation of a first-encounter greeting. "I'm fine. No problems at all." She has almost no short-term memory, the kind of problem a patient rarely is aware of, at least not in the beginning. It could come back in a flash, come back gradually, come back not at all. Otherwise, Jennie is the picture of health and passes every test.

Mirski is the attending neurointensivist this morning. He opens, "Hold up your hands for me . . . Good. Hold out a pizza box." This is one of the commoner lines in a neuro unit. The patient, usually half-sitting in bed, is to close her eyes and hold her hands palms up, at the same width apart as if she were holding out a pizza box. The team will look for signs that one arm or the other is drifting, or that the orientation of the palms is being lost—both measures of brain function at a primitive motor level, functions that lead to purposeful actions whose individual bits we do not need to think about. If you have been down in deep coma, going from "Wiggle your toes for me!" to "Can you close your eyes and hold out a pizza box?" marks major progress indeed.

This test is part of the neuro exam, among all the medical specialists the province of the neurologist. To Mirski, anesthesia taught him all the skills of intervention and rescue he would need for the NICU; after all, they had been crafted in the operating room. But it did not teach the critical diagnostic skills, the ability to see trouble down the road; for teaching that, he credits his neurology residency. The multipart neuro exam is the neurologist's way to get inside the patient's skull without scanner or saw. The brain, from its lowest stem to surface cortex, drives behavior. But more than that, the map of the pathways from cause to effect is wonderfully precise. Looking at simple behaviors, an experienced neurologist can infer what underlying brain tissue is damaged, at what level, and how extensively. As Mirski tells it, the entire neuro exam can be explained in 20 minutes, but it takes years to learn to read backward from the elicited behaviors to their causal roots.

It is the exclusive province of neurologists among physicians, but not exclusively theirs in this unit.

"Our nurses should be able to give a neuro exam better than a neurosurgeon," nurse manager Ski Lower says, "and, once their training is done, as well as a neurologist." That is not hyperbole to the neurointensivists. Mirski, discussing the enormous logistical problems they would face with the new, greatly enlarged unit, said equally flatly, "Nursing drives patient care. The nurses are with the patients around the clock."

In this Neuro ICU—uniquely, Mirski believes—the patient's nurse makes the first presentation on both morning and afternoon rounds. Presentation by each of the medical personnel is by system. Number one, of course, is neurological status. Observed changes, lab numbers, responses to medication, exam results, gut feelings. Two, cardiovascular system, including all the elements of hemodynamics from blood numbers to kidney function. Three, respiratory issues such as possible airway problems, ease of breathing. Four, GI and nutrition. Five, infectious diseases. Six, social issues such as family problems, personal needs.

To operate at this level requires never-ending training for the nurses. Orientation itself is long and demanding. There are classes covering respiratory and cardiac issues specific to neuroscience, on how to give the neuro exam, on the nature and consequences of AVMs, embolisms, and stroke, on the symptoms and problems in patients with Guillain-Barré syndrome. Nurses trained under Ski Lower's system must understand why medications are being administered, so they will be alert for both the expected results and possible adverse effects. And, as the unit is run by Mirski, nurses have to be informed of all medications and orders written by physicians.

Of the crises families face, especially in an intensive care unit, Lower says, "A doctor should never speak to a family about a patient's progress without a nurse present." Her reason is simple: from the moment doctors leave until they return again, family members will press the nurse for information, explanation, reinforcement, sometimes the plain-language translation of what they've just been told by a doctor.

Lower is interrupted in midsentence by today's resource nurse, trying to overcome a bed shortage. The nurse administrators as much as the intensivists control the logistics of patient movement in and out of the unit. She responds, "The patient in A on pentobarbital drip doesn't need to be here," if the numbers are such and such. "That might give you a little fluff tomorrow. But if the postops don't do well, that could take back your slack." Then jumps back into the question of training nurses.

For her, all of this has been a 20-year mission. It began when she became a nurse. She hated neuro at the outset, almost immediately went from hating to loving, and her life's work was born. She was hired here on October 13, 1981, to develop the nursing program for a neurosciences intensive care unit that was then just an idea. Over the years, she has developed a complex system of ranks and associated skills the nurses progress through, by classroom training, mentoring, and research. Like faculty, the nursing staff is self-governing, and everyone serves on governance committees and takes part in learning and mentoring.

She reads voraciously—management books, research, pop sociology about generational shifts—to help her deal with each new crop of her "baby nurses." Baby boomers, Gen X, Gen Y. She ticks off differences among the cohorts she has observed and studied, adapting strategies in order to make each feel part of the action. Her own children grown and her husband recently retired, she now spends a lot of days spreading the word at conferences. But Lower's drive is not directed simply to stumping for her causes. She has published voluminous research, sometimes coauthoring papers with the neurointensivists, sometimes writing on her own or with other nursing researchers—and those she trains are set on the same path.

"GOOD MORNING," Mirski repeats to Jennie Ray. Marie Stokes is her nurse as rounds begin, and it is she who reports that Jennie is making progress. It's sporadic, always an important qualifier here, but it is improvement. Stokes says, "She is confused at times as to date, sometimes as to place, but she's quickly reoriented." They discuss the "pop off" level of the intraventricular catheter. Like the escape valve on a steam kettle, this catheter valve is set to maintain a healthy amount of pressure in Jennie's ventricles. But if the pressure climbs above a safe limit, the valve will pop.

Jennie is also having vision problems that to a neurologist indicate she has had damage to her right optic tracts—toward the rear of her brain, not along the nerves' course from the eyes back to the middle brain. She has lost part of her left field of vision. That is, she can see out of both eyes, but it is the lower-left quadrant of the field of view in each eye that is knocked out. They anticipated the possibility of precisely that "field cut," given what they saw on her scans.

What the symptom tells them about the source of the problem derives from the complex route that light signals take from the eyes into the brain. The left and right optic nerves leave the retinas of their respective eyes carrying information from that eye only. They travel backward to a crossover point that is as major a landmark to a neurosurgeon as an interstate cloverleaf is to a pilot. That landmark is called the optic chiasm and makes the optic nerves resemble a large X as they travel from retinas to occipital lobes. Above the optic chiasm is the circle of Willis, and the pituitary gland's stalk dangles down over it, dropping from the hypothalamus. When the optic-nerve bundles cross over at the chiasm, they trade fibers. The bundles carrying the left visual field information from each eye travel to the right occipital lobe, at the rearmost part of the brain, and the right visual field information travels to the left occipital lobe. If the right fibers were cut at a certain point after the chiasm, the entire left visual field would have been lost, from each eye. Damaged farther back, at the calcarine fissure, a portion of the lower left quadrant is lost.

Blood or pressure from the hemorrhage has caused the disturbance to the optic nerve somewhere in that rear half of its course; it may be temporary and vanish completely if the pressure remains normal, providing Jennie does not have a new bleed. Or it could represent permanent damage. They still have not decided the best course of action to take for the AVM. Jennie seems alert enough this morning—chatty, amused by all the fuss, and certain she will be back on her feet and back to her studies in no time. It's hard to believe she had a brain hemorrhage a few days ago. Tamargo has offered the family several possibilities for treating the underlying problem. At the moment, it isn't clear which is best for Jennie Ray.

Rounds moves forward: Rita Serianni, A-comm ACA aneurysm clipping. Nurse Anna Madigan reads off her numbers. Rita is extending upward, meaning that if what should be a painful pressure is applied to her fingernail or breastbone, she does react against it—a good sign—but instead of grabbing for the offending hand, instinctively pushing or striking at it, she simply stretches her arm, the reaction coming out of her lower brain stem rather than the upper region, not a good sign. She opens her eyes when spoken to, which is good. Her family reports that at times she seems to follow and understand when they talk to her, and she sometimes smiles at their voices. She seems to be improving, a very good sign given all she has been through. Yesterday, in particular, she suffered from moderate to severe vasospasm, but she appears to have recovered from that as well. This morning she will have another transcranial Doppler test, one of the more interesting in the neurologist's toolbox.

Dr. Alex Razumovsky and Vlad Pomonorov are daily visitors to the NICU, pushing their computer cart laden with gadgets and wires. This is a tool straight out of a Tom Clancy thriller, miniaturized for the brain. In *The Hunt for Red October,* as Soviet and American submarines passed one another, sonar technicians heard the whoosh-whoosh of cavitation from the sub's propulsion screws. Pomorov will apply leads to several places on Rita Serianni's scalp, put on his headphones—there's an extra pair for visitors—and turn a few dials. He will listen to sounds just like those of the submarines, these pulses from blood coursing through blood vessels, coming and going, rising in frequency and dropping as he dials in target settings.

A train whistle blown as it approaches sounds higher in frequency than it does as the train recedes. That's the Doppler effect. Here, radio waves are pulsed into the patient's brain, and they bounce back from whatever structures they encounter, moving or stationary. The waves that strike moving targets—arterial blood, for example—return at a different frequency. The computer is programmed to seek and record the waves from the blood flowing through the arteries and veins of the brain. So the frequencies and volumes of the sounds Razumovsky and Pomorov hear reveal the identity of the arteries he has picked up. So far so good. But once Pomorov has identified one track sounding in his ears and dancing across the computer screen as the blood shooting through the middle cerebral artery he must record its velocity. That is the number the neurointensive team is after. If the artery is closing down in vasospasm, the blood will be moving at higher than normal pressure and velocity through the constricted space, just as water from a garden hose will shoot dozens of yards if the lip is closed over by a finger. Today, Rita Serianni's middle cerebral artery readings will not be normal, but they will be much better than yesterday's, and it was such a transcranial Doppler reading yesterday that confirmed her vasospasm in time to act against it successfully.

Mirski points out that they need to keep up the key numbers related to pressure in the brain—blood pressure, intracranial pressure, perfusion pressure—to counter vasospasm. But they don't want to challenge her arteries too much in the wake of her hemorrhage. Listening to him and the other intensivists and fellows on rounds, there often seems no link between patient care and research. Serianni's part in the IHAST2 study is over now. Yet the art applied daily, Mirski points out, works its way around solid landmarks—"best treatment" decisions, proven protocols—and those treatments, like the physicians who apply them, are in every sense driven by research.

Days pass and, one by one, the three women who had little in common except hemorrhagic stroke and at different times the same Neurointensive Care address, leave the unit for the floor, not healed but out of crisis. First Jennie Ray, then Donna Soja, finally Rita Serianni. Their stories' conclusions would be as different as their beginnings.

Drive, drive, drive, all related but no two meanings quite the same. Singular yet hardly ever occurring unmixed and elemental, almost always in a complex. You can imagine schematizing each drive as a different melodic line on a scale, one ripping strong and fast, darting high and low, and another slow, measured, not loud – now and then resonating with the first. Then a third line somewhere between them. Put them all together and they reflect in one another, a powerful multipart synergy—when everything works and there are no clashes or conflicts, of course. But in harmony or cacophony, the elements of drive are never simple.

CHAPTER 10

Labyrinths

ERE IS DAN HANLEY, tall, silver-haired, at 52 the image of the accomplished Johns Hopkins neuroscience physician and pioneer that he is, returned to the research that started his academic career. He has a serious demeanor and no-nonsense attitude toward peers and subordinates, but shows an engaging, self-deprecating sense of humor all the same. Slow and deliberate in speaking, carefully forming his words. He is an intent believer in *thought process* in medicine, in the global reach of problems and thus a required global thinking to find solutions. He is glad if you pick up on a proferred thought, quick to correct if you do not take it in the right direction.

Like other hard-driving intensivists in this story, much of his thrust was parental. He hails from

Maine, son and namesake of a widely admired and recently deceased physician who distinguished himself in a career of civilian medicine and as a combat physician with the Tenth Mountain Division in World War II. It was Daniel F. Hanley, Sr. who spurred the drive to identify Olympic athletes using banned steroids and other performance-enhancing drugs. Now the son is a full professor with an endowed chair, and he is as soft-spoken as one of his favorite mentors remembers him as a resident. But he has a hot temper, and it flares at the same thinking that always hit his hot button.

Here is its essence:

It is one of Hanley's first nights on call at Johns Hopkins as a new assistant professor and ICU neurologist. First case, first crisis. The emergency room had a man with an intraventricular hemorrhage and wanted to know if Hanley would admit him to critical care. Of course, he said.

Blood in the ventricles was a deadlier sign then than it is now. Tear an artery within the ventricles and blood pumps hard into the inter-connected cisterns, making them swell, compressing and perhaps crushing the delicate surrounding brain tissue. That's bad enough in the region outside, say, the lateral ventricles. They are surrounded by the cerebrum, where the brain thinks, speaks, hears, touches, sees. But blow out the bottom cistern—the fourth ventricle—and there goes control of heartbeat and breathing, the animal functions that mark not human life but life itself. At that time, intraventricular hemorrhage was considered the point at which you could offer no treatment to a patient, because there was no chance for survival. That, at least, was the received wisdom.

As a result, because he had admitted this patient, Hanley immediately came into direct confrontation with a senior neurosurgeon.

An intraventricular hemorrhage is fatal, the neurosurgeon pointed out. So why would anyone take up a precious, life-saving critical-care bed with an IVH victim whose brain was already killed? _Why are you wasting this bed with someone who is sure to die when it could hold a person I might save?_

Hanley argued that this hemorrhage victim could be saved, that if the blood were drained neurosurgically, shunted out, this case . . . But he got nowhere. The neurosurgeon had no intention of operating on a lost cause, creating a vegetable instead of a fatality. That emergency faded into the next. Hanley doesn't know the outcome of the case, but "in all likelihood, he died." The only way to have proved his point would have been to save the patient.

Hanley's war, as always, is against nihilism, that fairly common term of disparagement among doctors. Nihilists of the twentieth century's pessimistic Lost Generation saw life as meaningless, therefore argued that there was no point in doing or believing anything. As used here, the term has lost none of its negative connotation, but "nothing" has become quite relative. To Hanley, the neurosurgeon of his confrontation was a nihilist, choosing to do nothing, because the patient would die anyway, rather than trying to save him. To that neurosurgeon, of course, he was nothing of the kind. He was saving those who could be saved, not squandering resources on those who could not be, which would be sentimentalist. But today's combatant against nihilism—Columbia's Stephan Mayer, say, working around the clock to save the patient everyone has written off—can emerge as tomorrow's nihilist, urging that _this_ patient be allowed the dignified death she pleaded for.

Hanley uses the term _nihilist_ more often than most as he discusses his concepts of research and its purposes, of intensive care and its purposes. Aren't the outcomes of IVH's usually fatal? he was once asked. "The _presumed_ outcome is fatal," he shot back. "Sometimes when we presume the outcome is fatal, and give up, it becomes fatal. If you're on a ventilator and unconscious, and we decide not to do anything and take you off the ventilator, then you have a pretty high likelihood of dying, which will prove you had a fatal attack."

Whether you are looking at cardiac arrest, ischemic stroke or intraventricular hemorrhage— and he studies them all—the question remains the same. Take a group of patients with a very low chance of survival, who might be written off as goners. Is there not some subset within that actually has good odds of survival, with proper treatment? This, of course, is one of the fundamental questions not only of medical research but in clinical treatment. It's a critical question for oncologists reviewing their patients' prognoses, in an effort to separate out those who might benefit from aggressive treatment from those who would go through the agony for nothing, when palliative care is what they need. It's the question asked by cardiologists treating heart attack victims, to determine who will benefit from what degree of aggressive treatment. Hanley applies that question often. The phrase "identify that subset of patients amenable to treatment . . . " pops up continually in his discourse.

And significantly, Hanley's defining memories of himself in action in the past, from student to attending physician to neurointensive leader, are anchored in combat with *nihil*. Single combat with death. He had a moment of epiphany, when the direction of his career became clear even before he saw particular pathways.

The year was 1978. He was completing an internal medicine residency at Cornell Medical School in Manhattan and simultaneously studying pain and neuropharmacology on a fellowship in neurology at neighboring Memorial Sloan-Kettering. He liked neurology—the thought process, the intricacies of the brain. "But I did not like all neurologists. It bothered me that there weren't so many real things to do for the patient." He particularly admired Jerome Posner, as did his mentors and peers. Until recently, the great unknown of neuroscience had been encapsulated in one word, *coma*. To physicians, coma had meant pretty much what it means to most people: zero, blackness, the unarticulated lack of brain activity that was a step from death and from which few returned. Then, in 1965, Fred Plum, head of neurology at Cornell, and Posner had written the book that marked a revolution in neurology: *Stupor and Coma*. Now coma was no longer a single blackness to residents like Hanley, it was a complex gradation between death and full consciousness. With works such as that in hand and the development of the Glasgow Coma Scale a few years later, it now became realistic to ask, *Can we identify a subset of comatose patients amenable to treatment?*

One night Hanley was resident on call for neurology, and one of his patients was dying. He determined to bring the man back and grappled over the next two days, nonstop, without sleep, with all the tools and skills he could muster, back and forth, morning through night. And in the middle of the second night the man died, just like that. Hanley was sitting there—maybe it was the next morning—feeling like hell, miserable, depressed, and Posner came up to him. Hanley remembers his words vividly. *You did a good job with that patient. You kept him alive for as long as possible. Not everyone can do that. You're good at it. You should consider doing that.*

Spurred on, Hanley completed his medicine residency and headed off to a second, in neurology, at Johns Hopkins. He recalls another particularly admired role model from those years, Allan Ropper, a year ahead of him at Cornell. "Allan taught me a new standard about clinical treatment," he says. And for his part, Allan Ropper says Plum and Posner's book and views helped shaped his life, as well. In fact, that led him directly into neurological intensive care, for which he not only created the first unit but wrote the first text. "There is nothing more fascinating than coma," Ropper says now. Who could have thought such a thing a generation ago?

All these years later, Posner does not recall the encounter Hanley so vividly remembers—but he is glad to be remembered for his good words. Avuncular in manner, incisive in comment, he says, "I wasn't always so kind." He remembers Hanley well—"bright, eager, articulate" as well as soft-spoken. But the lesson Posner takes from the episode is that Hanley "probably learned more from those two days than from any other two weeks" of training, and such a learning experience in residency "could never happen again." Work hours for residents now are strictly limited by law, and after a shift they are required to leave the hospital. The change has been widely hailed, and widely criticized. But it was in that demanding climate that Hanley developed his own demanding sense of patient care, carried to whatever lengths it must be to win or lose.

Soon Hanley stood on the roof of Johns Hopkins and saw Baltimore and the bay spread out around him, and thought about new ways to treat the brain-injured patients below. The idea of a specialty intensive care unit for neuro patients was not new. In fact, it was a logical extension of the movement toward specialization and subspecialization that swept through the sciences for most of the twentieth century and was reflected in medical education and research, though the tide would turn in medicine by the mid-nineties. It was only in 1969 that Johns Hopkins had established a Neurology Department, joining a small number of academic medical centers that had done so earlier. Guy McKhann, its founding chair, wrote years later that before then, neurology services usually had been attached to internal medicine, sometimes psychiatry.

But, Hanley noted, large institutions rarely accomplish major undertakings in a single, smooth action, and steps were taken forward and back in the Neuro ICU arena, but the demand for more critical-care beds for neurosurgery patients set the final stage. "It became obvious that the bottleneck for neurosurgery was not the OR, but the ICU," he said. In October

1981 the Neurology Department persuaded Ski Lower to leave Washington Hospital Center, where she managed the trauma and open-heart unit, and come to Hopkins to create a specialty nursing program for neurointensive care. When Hanley joined the faculty in July 1983, Neurosurgery chair Donlin Long, Anesthesia chair Mark Rogers and McKhann picked him to build the foundation of a new subspecialty to run that unit. Soon after, anesthesiologist Cecil Borel was named codirector.

Most of the country's new Neuro ICUs were run by neurosurgeons, because nearly all of the patients in need of intensive care at that time were either heading into or coming out of neurosurgery. Neurosurgery's Long didn't want that, and he was, by all accounts, rare in his willingness to surrender control of the Neuro ICU. His reasoning, as he offers it, is clear. "If we have top-flight neurointensivists who can manage our patients, we can spend more time in the operating room." The other side of the coin, however, is that the neurosurgery residents being trained to understand and respond to the sequellae—the consequences—of their surgeries would now be working under someone *other than a neurosurgeon*. Few neurosurgery chairs were willing to let go.

Turned loose to create their unit, Hanley and Borel moved quickly, and within a few years had established one of the largest units in the country run entirely by neurointensive care specialists, whom they were training or had trained and kept on as attendings. Soon graduates were either starting up or taking over the operation of neuro units from Quebec to California. Most new programs called for a one-year fellowship. Johns Hopkins demanded two: fellows would spend half their time carrying out the research into the intensive care of the injured brain that would be the underpinnings of this "evidence-based medicine"; and they would spend half their time in the unit, with Hanley and Borel and Lower and the new-minted neurointensive nurses. Two decades later, Hanley's CV lists no fewer than 13 trainees who have gone on to direct or codirect NICUs, roughly a third of the 40 or 50 truly specialized units in the country. And, Allan Ropper says, "Dan Hanley brought a real academic rigor and respect to neurointensive care."

But he was also the administrator of a hospital unit, and units need constant funding. The NICU was growing, so it needed growing funding from both public and private sources. Other neurointensivist mentors struggled, as Hanley did, to find fellowship money and seed money for major grant applications that would bring in research dollars. Neurology Departments, to put it crassly but realistically, are not hospital profit centers. Anesthesiology is, but that was not Hanley's primary home. Still, he struggled more successfully than most. Because the Johns Hopkins NICU is "closed," only neurointensivists can be in charge of patient care in the unit. That emphasis is important for two reasons. First, the idea was to create a cadre of specialists who could manage the whole patient, not just consult on their own subspecialty. Second, that meant there had to be enough of them to cover the entire unit. That, in turn, meant still more money—for training, overhead, faculty salaries.

For all his academic prowess, though, Hanley's reputation grew most as a clinician. And talking to him now, it's plainly where his heart was. *Rescue.*

"I have seen him weep, many times, in frustration over losing a patient," Anish Bhardwaj recalls, as does Ski Lower. But Lower also recalls a Dan Hanley who could not let go when it was past time to do so. "He has his miracle rescues, there is no doubt about that," she says. "But I remember times when families had to persuade him it was time to let go, when I knew it was *long* past time."

Nothing ever looks the same from inside as out—trite but true. As everywhere, retrospectively watching the growth of the concept and the concrete reality of the neurointensivist yields two different stories, depending on perspective, complementary to one another at some points, snapping neatly together like puzzle pieces, at other points seeming unrelated.

Hanley and Lower are like siblings, one intensivist says; joined at the hip, says another. But like many people in tight partnerships at close quarters, sparks flew, sometimes furiously, over many years, between the neurologist developing the idea of a neurointensivist-managed NICU and the nurse who, perhaps more than any other anywhere, developed the idea of the *nurse* as the key to managing the NICU patient.

When Hanley, a brand-new assistant professor fired up by his own dedication and training, as well as by the ideas put forth by Ropper, Posner, and others, was given the charge to create a Neurosciences Critical Care Unit, the possibilities were endless—for achievement and for conflict. Several of the long-time hands in the unit paint the same picture of the early years. Lower alone is happy to have her name signed to it.

From the start, she says, the unit never got support from Neurology, not the kind it needed to accomplish what it had to. Why not? First, maybe, because only Hanley, Borel, and Lower believed it could succeed. One NICU faculty member says, "I honestly believe that those in Neurology thought Dan was doomed to failure."

For his part, Hanley speaks nothing but praise for McKhann, right from the unit's founding. McKhann himself says he and everyone concerned gave it all the support they could, and that Hanley's proving the concept entailed even more evolving support.

Second, for Lower, even in the traditional academic setting of Johns Hopkins, Neurology stood out as focused on "research, research, research." That meant physicians' exhausting clinical duties—*saving patients*—counted far less in their evaluations for promotion and other advancement than did success in landing grants. This last is a complaint that can be heard to varying degrees from faculty throughout academic medicine—in fact, throughout all academia, where "Publish or perish" has been the rule since time immemorial. To realize his vision, Hanley was always on the hunt for philanthropy, right from the start, without rest, Lower and others say. For his own part, Hanley counts his ability to bring in funds among his strengths in building the unit, crediting Borel for his skill in day-to-day administration and personnel management.

And it's worth noting how different the views of the "academic imperative" can be with changed perspective—like that of McKhann, the founding chair of the Neurology Department who now researches Alzheimer's and other diseases at Hopkins's Zanvyl Krieger Mind Brain Institute. He says that, at a hospital like Johns Hopkins, clinical care should drive physicians toward research. It's not that patient care should be anything but the best, "but it is not enough," he says. "We must always be asking how we can do it better. That's a research question."

Then there were conflicts over that founding vision—for starters, between Hanley and Lower. Conflicts so sharp, she says, that shortly after the unit's opening, she and Hanley were no longer talking to one another at all. They communicated only through their secretaries.

One day, Lower found herself scheduled for lunch at a French restaurant downtown, but her secretary kept dodging about with whom, only repeating that it was important. It was a trick. Hanley's secretary had done the same. There they were, face-to-face over lunch. And face-to-face, they hammered out their differences.

For several years after that day, "nursing never had a better friend than Dan Hanley," Lower says. "He not only supported us in the unit, he went to bat for us with other units. It certainly didn't get him any Mr. Popularity award." NICU nursing never could have flourished to achieve what it has today without Hanley, she says. "No question about it."

Soon the NICU had grown: 4 beds became 8, then 12 and 16. Fellows came aboard—like Mike Diringer, recommended by Ropper because at the time Ropper had no fellowships and, somehow, Hanley did. There were four Johns Hopkins fellows a year—two junior, two senior—meaning four salaries and overhead budgets. And although the success of the concept and the unit was being proved, to those in it, there was never more than middling financial support from their "half-time" home department of Neurology, Anesthesia being the other half. All that Marek Mirski will say of this period, when he was a resident, fellow and, at the end, new junior faculty, is to point out that Neurology is always a cash-poor department, everywhere. Neurologists are funded by their consultations, which may fluctuate. But in addition, as we've heard, neurologists tend to be—pun aside—more cerebral, and Mirski says carelessness about billing is commonplace in Neurology departments everywhere. By contrast, he says, Anesthesia is a department of well-defined, critical procedures that go on, as the OR and ICUs do, around the clock.

In any case, Lower says, for Hanley the constant hunt for resources and budget became obsessive. So did his secrecy about finances. "I told him, Dan, you're going to lose the support of your own people if you don't open up with them." But finances remained his business and his worry alone.

To some of those Hanley trained, as well as to Lower and others he worked with, along with the obsession to maintain the unit's resources came an obsessive control of its physicians' activities. It was in the second decade of the unit that Lower saw a crisis coming. By the mid-nineties, the man who was the best friend nursing ever had had lost the support of nursing. "My nurses were ready to quit," Lower says. "We were faced with the destruction of the unit itself."

That's one side of the story, leading to an inevitable breach.

The other: "I don't think I was or am very controlling," Hanley says. "But maybe I'd agree that I am. If controlling means taking a vision and creating a reality where no one else ever had then or has since, then I guess I'm controlling. If you want to create something new and important with limited resources, then you must be in charge. You have to limit the degrees of freedom with which people operate." That phrase, "limit the degrees of freedom," from the statistical analysis used in medical research, brings anger from some, including Lower. "I think you need to do the opposite," she says.

Others became angered because they felt Hanley did not share credit for the unit's successes—including the patient rescues—or that he failed to give proper publication credit to junior faculty who needed it most. The complaints may sound, to an outsider, either damning or petty, depending on viewpoint—perhaps were each, by turns. But they are routinely familiar as the tinder that often, incrementally over time, consumes administrators from medicine to science to government to the largest corporations.

John Ulatowski, who trained under Hanley and then became a senior faculty member and attending physician, has recently moved out of clinical care and into administrative roles at the hospital. He will say nothing of the whole period. But he points out, "Nothing is created without the individual willing to be the pioneer. But often there comes a time when that isn't the right person to run things anymore." And of Marek Mirski's selection as Hanley's replacement, "We made the right choice."

Hanley firmly believes that it was the success of the Neuro ICU that angered many outside it, and that it was the views of those outside, and one or two within, that led the new Neurology chair, John Griffin, to ask him to step down. Not without a fight, he wouldn't, but after a fight, he did.

A couple of years earlier, Hanley had taken a sabbatical, during which he studied, taught and shared ideas with his counterpart NICU specialists in Heidelberg, Germany. Many say that European, and especially German, critical care is far ahead of America's. Hanley is convinced of it, after spending a year with Werner Hacke, considered the leading name in German neurological intensive care.

Hanley returned certain of new directions for the unit. After he stepped down, he took ideas he had developed for bringing the brain back after illness or trauma and he turned them into a new career direction, as holder of the Legum Chair in Neurology's new division of Brain Injury Outcomes.

MEDICINE AS SCIENCE represents experiment, measurement, and conclusion, observation upon observation; clumps of observations reproduced a hundredfold, catalogued and built into hypotheses and protocols. Medicine as art represents an exquisite balancing of opposites, a willingness to deal with contradictions; sometimes to suspend forebodings, at others to heed them; sometimes to suspend pragmatism in favor of optimism, at others to finally lay down the weapons and let go.

The science and the art do not always mix well. Sometimes they war, in the same physicians bent over the same patient. But in all cases, the art and science have this goal in common: by careful, prepared, repeated observation of thousands of slight variations, to avoid surprise. To find the stable points within chaos, which means control. To maintain stability and balance. At the same time to avoid that other stability, the end of turbulence, the settling into terminal order, which is death.

Intensive care, like emergency medicine, integrates the art and science under extreme conditions. Surprise is regular, death happens. Each person spiraling down toward oblivion is a whole new learning experience, for the leader of other leaders, down to the newest fellow. But in some memorable cases all the relief and terror dance out in a terrible string. Every success leads to failure and every failure, re-righted, inverts to success, toggling. The exit from one labyrinth that brings a flush of relief only marks the entrance to a new maze. Labyrinths nested like Russian dolls—but this time no two are quite the same, so the secrets learned in one offer only hints for dealing with the next.

Wednesday, November 7, 1990

E L L E N   A P P L E   H E A R S   Jack get up around 7 and go into the bathroom, as usual, to get ready for their morning walk before work. And as usual she allows herself a few extra minutes to come around before following him. Although they are new to Baltimore from Pittsburgh, where they'd spent most of their adult lives, Jack still is the top salesman for London Fog apparel. He just wanted a new territory; she has switched from teaching to consulting for an educational testing company. Both are enjoying the change. His boss boasts that Jack Apple has sold more raincoats than anyone else in the world, but if true, it's not something that turns Jack's head. Jack and Ellen are as down-to-earth as they come. Still, they have few friends here and their three grown children are scattered, though, happily, they remain a close family. The events leading to the Gulf War are brewing in the Middle East, according to the late news just before they turned in, and in the midterm congressional elections just yesterday . . .

Was any of this going through Ellen's mind as the familiar sounds of morning arose in her senses? She has no recollection. It was the beginning of the kind of routine day you take for granted until the routine vanishes in a puff, quickly taking on a magical, retrospective glow as you realize you may never know it again.

After minutes went by Ellen realized there was no rustling of Jack in the closet, dressing, picking out a shirt, riffling through ties. She popped up. There he sat in the chair, holding his head.

"What's wrong?"

"I have the worst headache I've ever had." He looked gray, even green, and was sweating profusely. Jack had been diabetic for 20 years, though it had always been well controlled. She ran downstairs for orange juice, to counter the symptoms, but after taking a few sips he went back into the bathroom and vomited.

The next events are a blur: she talks to Jack's doctor's receptionist, but the doctor is at the hospital already. She helps Jack into their sedan. He needs a hand but says he's okay except for the headache.

The nightmare intrudes slowly. By the time she has edged onto Cross Country Boulevard, traffic has slowed in the rushhour; it crawls by Falls Road, nears gridlock on Interstate 87 south toward Baltimore and Johns Hopkins. She has made many choices this morning, feeling her way for the right ones. She did not call 911, knowing they would take Jack to the *nearest* hospital. She wanted him in Johns Hopkins, where his doctor was at this moment. She is a stranger to these highways, so has little idea of the best way downtown at this hour. But she knows where Hopkins is, exiting toward it at Fayette, by now terrified. Hours seem to have gone by, and Jack has gone from speaking slowly to slumped in silence, unconscious. She had to stop several times so he could throw up. Now he doesn't seem to be breathing.

And the coup de grâce: Lying between them and rescue in the medical center looming ahead are the chaotically twisting ramparts of construction zones, where streets suddenly become one-way run into streets that have always been one-way. The cavernous tunnel of Baltimore's new subway line is inching toward its last stop at Johns Hopkins Hospital, leaving the entire surface world like a war zone. The citadel is right before her. There is no way to it. No way. She has to stop as Jack rouses to vomit again. She asks directions. *Turn right here,* a workman tells her. Down a blind alley. Ask again. *Right, then two blocks, left* . . . Around and around the hospital she drives, sometimes spinning out farther away, never getting to the emergency room.

In near panic she realizes that the one sure way *in* would simply be to drive the car into a pole. The police would come and take them to the emergency room.

Somehow at last she reaches the emergency room, parks, and rushes inside. Seconds later she, an ER nurse, and a security guard rush back pushing a wheelchair, the guard saying over and over *you cannot park your car here, not even for a minute, not even for a second.* But the two take Jack inside, and Ellen again plows into the welter of construction and under-ground excavation, into never-neverland in the hunt for hospital parking. Still, Jack is inside. Everything will be fine now.

But the hours bring bad news. Jack may have had a brain hemorrhage. He has been drifting farther and farther away. He looks up at her. The doctor asks Jack his wife's name. Jack looks at Ellen and says, "Shirley Apple." When she says no, he says, "Susan." The nightmare is full-blown.

Inside, Jack Apple's brain is on the brink of devastation, but unlike the sort of hemorrhage that shows a great dark blob on a CT scan that anyone can spot, his requires an experienced eye just to see, and a mind trained deeply and well to understand.

The branching trees of the great brain arteries spread from the trun-klike base to the outermost crown to nourish every small cluster of cells that underlie us, tracing evolution's route from the primitive brain stem— ours remarkably similar to those of lower mammals, which are not vastly different from those of lizards—upward into the powerful, ancient diencephalon, ever higher and outward into the enfolding sheet of the cortex. The six-layered cortex that spreads and crumples over its spheroidal four lobes provides the visual image of the brain we all recognize instantly. The "higher" brain is what we think of as distinctly human.

There's justification for thinking this way. The stretch from a smart ape to a Shakespeare, Bach, or Einstein is probably measured in this square meter of six-deep neurons folded up into the braincase. Within the neurons' connections are the secrets of great hunters, of farmers who can build surpluses into wealth, of city builders and medical miracle workers. In sum, within this square meter lie our gifts. But it is the old, deep structures that are life itself. First comes the brain stem, its swelled medulla oblongata with the large pons appearing to be strapped around it, then, above, the bundles of neuronal relays and mediators of the midbrain and diencephalon, all buried deeply within that cauliflower cap. These most vital structures can best be seen by exploring the brain from within, as swimmers through a series of upward reaching caves rather than climbers crawling around on the dome.

In here is where Jack Apple's problem lies. Rising up from just ahead of the brain stem is that series of cisterns, the ventricles, so often a major topic in neuro medicine. As the cisterns rise into the upper brain, they spread left and right, looking, on brain scans, like moose-antler shaped caverns in the middle of each cerebral hemisphere. The cerebrospinal fluid, whose pressure is so closely watched, is made in specialized structures embedded in the ventricle walls; the CSF not only protects the brain, cushioning its center, it carries away dead cells and used-up metabolites.

The cisterns are named from top to bottom. At base, the swollen tube of the fourth ventricle comes between the brain stem in front and the cerebellum aft. Moving upward, the third ventricle, if its walls were clear, would offer views to the fore of the large left and right thalami, along with the hypothalami forming the diencephalon. The third ventricle's ceiling is hugged by the left and right hippocampi, crucial for storing and recalling memories. Upward from the third vent, through the canal called the foramen of Monro, we reach the great caverns of the left and right lateral ventricles, each with separate grottoes marking their intrusion into the upper brain. Each has a horn into the temporal lobe and another horn reaching into the frontal lobe.

Ischemic damage in the brain is localized: whichever center depends on the lost arterial flow is "out." But events in these cisterns are not localized, for the ventricles touch everywhere in the brain at once, and they press from within. We've heard how dangerous their swelling can be, but, even before pressure damages the fundament, slight changes ripple throughout the human personality—the ability to see, to talk, to understand what is being said, to make that final leap, *I see.* These milder effects can be transient and no more cause for alarm than that name on the tip of your tongue that won't come, or they can be harbingers of far worse to come, a mild tremor before the cataclysm.

The doctors in the NICU told Ellen they suspected an aneurysm had leaked but needed to confirm it with an angiogram tomorrow. If they were right, Jack should undergo neurosurgery to have the aneurysm clipped before it re-bled or burst. Meanwhile, they told her all the risks: death, stroke, loss of motor skills. When Ellen first saw Jack in the unit, "there was almost no place to touch him," what with the IV in his arm, blood pressure monitor line, central line to monitor his heart, oxygen into his nose, temporary catheter-drain relieving pressure in his skull.

Somewhere in this ventricular territory, far outward from the circle of Willis in a place that would never be found, a small artery had swelled, leaving Jack clutching his head in agony. Brain tissue has no feeling, but blood vessels are very sensitive to pressure. And then, in the bedroom or on the drive here, the vessel had bled through the wall of the left lateral ventrical and sent caustic blood into the cerebrospinal fluid of the giant cistern, pumping up the pressure.

By midnight, back at home, the Apples' children had arrived: Doug, 30; Betsy, 28; Linda, 26. Friends had gathered who would support Ellen through the worst, and as sometimes happens, she found they had more and better friends than they had known. A call to the Neuro ICU: Jack was stable. "We talked and cried and went to bed," Ellen wrote in the journal she decided to keep, to provide focus and stabilizing routine.

The next day, it was as though a terrible storm had blown in and as quickly dissipated, leaving her to wonder if she had imagined or at least exaggerated the severity of the situation. Jack was awake and alert. When the kids showed up, he asked why they had come. He was fine. Sort of. He asked why everyone appeared double. He couldn't remember the events of the day before at all. He fidgeted and talked incessantly. From semiconscious, he had now "become a person who couldn't shut up." But he knew Ellen again, his mind was intact. The road back didn't seem much of a stretch.

"We laughed and joked with him and were amazed that he had progressed so much in such a short time," she wrote that evening.

Michael Williams, then a neurointensivist fellow in the NICU, answered all her questions. The fluid pressure in Jack's brain had stretched or compressed nerves and tissues within the skull. That led to double vision and memory loss. Now, with the fluid being drained, the intensivists needed to watch for further bleeding.

They were nearly out of the woods. Doug Apple brought his father a *New York Times,* and Jack read and commented unhappily on a report that 200,000 more troops were heading for the Persian Gulf. Betsy asked if reading made his head hurt. "[President] Bush makes my head hurt," he shot back, to a round of laughter. And then he took off on the craziness of Daryl Strawberry's getting more than $20 million to play baseball. He balked at wearing the pressurized leggings used to keep blood pressure constant in bedridden patients. They were hot and uncomfortable. But, Betsy said, they're contributing to your overall well-being, to getting better. Just believe it, she said. "Daddy, make a leap of faith." "Leap of faith!" he cried. "I can't leap with these things on." Onward!

Crash. A bad Friday night. That was the word from the hospital when Ellen called first thing Saturday morning. Agitated and sometimes delirious, Jack had tried to pull his tubes out. It had taken four people to restrain him and they finally had to bind his wrists with heavy leather straps.

Why? Perhaps vasospasm. So *did* he have a stroke? Almost certainly, given what would unfold, but never proven. Stroke refers to the infarction—death—of any brain tissue as a result of oxygen deprivation. This was still the period when most doctors thought that the initial "insult" to the brain either killed cells or didn't. If the cells were dead, that was a stroke and that was that. Those who argued that stroke should be treated as an emergency got little support. What was the emergency? The stricken tissue was dead or alive and there was nothing to offer but restful care— palliative treatment—during slow recovery.

By 1990 it was becoming clear to specialists that the process of brain cell death from stroke is very complicated, with weeks of latent effects. What looked like quick damage they were discovering to be a slow, subterranean process. And there, of course, lay opportunity. If you could bring those blurry events into sharp focus, you might intervene. And if you could intervene, then you could prevent the events from continuing.

We've seen hemorrhagic strokes, but ischemic strokes, in which arteries are blocked but not ruptured, are far more common. They can be caused by an embolism, a "boulder" blocking the arterial pipe, say a bit of calcified cholesterol that breaks off an artery wall and travels upward until it washes into a vessel too narrow for it to pass. Ischemic strokes can also be caused by thrombosis, in which the clot buildup takes place right in the wall of the brain artery, eventually narrowing so blood flows at a trickle or stops altogether.

With ventricular pressure causing vessels to clamp down in Jack's head, he lost touch with where he was and even his own condition as the frontal-lobe centers that "put it all together" lost oxygen. From the first, the intensivists pushed back into the arteries with fluids to keep up the blood supply—risky since he'd already bled—and with salts to draw water out of the brain tissue, along with the drain aimed at keeping down the swelling. The strategy, and sedation, seemed to work. He was almost out of intensive care. He was calm and sleepy all day. Slowly, up he came. By Monday, Ellen was able to write in praise of her children's strength and persistence in getting and understanding information in what seemed denouement. "I have been so pleased with the care he is receiving and the communicativeness of the medical staff. They answer all our questions so patiently." She was prepared to see him next in a regular room, on the upward road.

Then, reversal. "What a day today has been!" she wrote on Tuesday. By afternoon, Jack was tubed and wired again. And out of it again. This time it was ventriculitis, they said, inflammation of the ventricles. The cistern walls in the center of the brain are never supposed to come in contact with the outer world. For nearly a week, Jack's had been open through the tube inserted to relieve CSF pressure, and no matter how sterile conditions are made, there is often a way in for microbes. The doctors hit the infection with powerful antibiotics; but "powerful" cuts two ways. The toxins that take out microbes also can damage the kidneys and liver and the delicate, hairlike cilia of the inner ear that are responsible for hearing and balance.

But by 5 p.m. Jack was "up" again, teasingly asking daughter Betsy why she was wearing his favorite sweater, naming its Italian designer without a hitch in fluency. At 7:30 he was sitting in a chair for the first time in a week, surprising them and Laurel Moore, another neurointensivist fellow. Mother and daughter left him in the evening sitting in a chair reading *Business Week,* and for once found him not awfully different next day.

But against the backdrop of his improved physical appearance and all that has been restored, Ellen sees how profound the change has been. Jack can repeat what is said to him by the neurologists. He can respond correctly to questions. But he cannot express *himself.* She wrote, "He could not express his thoughts. They either did not come, or came out as completely unrelated words or even nonsense words."

The original problem now seems compounded by a round of vasospasm, and his doctors fear it will kill him if they do not act. They can infer which arteries have been clamped, and thus which brain centers are starving for oxygen, by what Jack cannot do.

He has no trouble forming and speaking words. That indicates no damage to the brain's "speech-motor" focus, called Broca's area. Broca's lies along the side of the frontal lobe. If you picture the brain viewed from the side as a boxing glove and the temporal lobe its fat thumb, Broca's lies right about where the thumb tucks into the "padded" frontal lobe, and it is continuous with the rest of the motor control region that runs in a strip upward across the brain over the top, down into the middle of the hemishere, usually the left one. The motor strip is just ahead of the valley that marks the front-rear divide of frontal and parietal lobes.

Jack also has no problems understanding what is said to him, which would indicate damage to the speech-comprehension region. Called

Wernicke's area, it lies a few inches back from Broca's area, on the top rear of the temporal lobe, right where that imagined thumb joins the heel of the boxing glove. Just as Broca's speech-production area is near the motor strip, Wernicke's area adjoins the auditory center, which lies just above the temporal lobe. It makes sense that related areas should lie near one another, but such physical proximity is not a rule in the brain.

Much of Jack's comprehension, responsive action, and articulation showed working frontal lobes. But in those frontal lobes, where our "own thoughts" arise, connections were not being made correctly to the speech areas. Jack knew what he wanted to say. He could form and speak words. But he could not speak the words he wanted.

If the doctors simply waited, odds were that the oxygen-starved regions of Jack's forebrain would become ischemic from having no oxygen, and they would die. The only way out they could recommend was angioplasty, a technique then new for brain arteries, developed and performed successfully against heart vasospasm.

First they would image the arteries of Jack's brain with an angiogram. That was somewhat risky because it involved putting dye in a major artery that would provide a real-time picture of the brain's blood flow. It was best done now while he was medically on the upswing. They would find the constricted vessel, then snake a thin catheter through all the twists and turns to the constriction. Reaching it, they would open a tiny balloon at the catheter tip, press the balloon through the constriction, and break the strangulation.

Ellen, children, friends prepared a sophisticated list of questions:

"Do vasospasms spread to other arteries?"

They don't appear to spread, but they do tend to be systemic. So one may be a harbinger of others.

"How many arteries can be done" with angioplasty?

It depends on how diffuse the vasospasm area is. It's pretty common for two arteries to be opened at once this way, but sometimes more are done if the angiogram shows that's needed.

"If one [artery] is opened, does it open others?"

No, but the most common situation involves one artery.

"How risky is balloon angioplasty?"

Only four had been done so far at Hopkins. One patient had improved enormously; two had stayed the same; one had died. Not good odds, but better, the doctors said, than the alternative.

Ellen and Betsy decided to okay the procedure. They held hands in the waiting room, sobbing, wondering if their decision would save or kill him. They decided to go for the saving procedure and not look back in regret, no matter what.

Jack was for it, and that helped. Awake and alert now, he said, "Let's get on with it," as he waited through the tedious, cumbersome procedure of having his IV stand and monitor rack prepared for "takeoff" as he was moved to a gurney for transport into the basement, then a hundred yards or more down that gloomy, gun-metal gray corridor to the radiology suite where the angiography would be performed.

And two hours later, back the procession came, buoyant and enthused. No vasospasm had been found. That was good news.

"He is much better today," Ellen wrote of the day after, "sitting up and talking with us, remembering people in great detail . . . . "

She remembered especially the nurses. Kathy Murphy: "She tells us everything in such great detail—talking to her is as good as talking to the doctors . . . " Inez Wendel, on the 3–11 shift, "has been fantastic . . ." Ken Norris "also rates high."

Then: Today "he was eating by rote, using a fork for soup, not really knowing what he was doing . . . "

And: "Today was awful. Jack is completely unresponsive and unable to find words or even answer simple questions . . . He could not identify his wedding ring by name or tell time. He didn't know what city he used to live in . . . He doesn't seem happy to see us—just off in his own quiet, unconnecting world."

Mike Williams believed this was temporary, that the fluid balance still had to be achieved but that no permanent damage had been done. Fluid pressure squeezed down on this normal brain, and suddenly a man could not speak or put a thought together. Pressure relieved, he would be back to normal—a graphic reminder of what we are, at bottom. Off, on, off, on. Ellen writes: "Mardi, his nurse tonight, tries to reassure us that this is the way it is . . . It is so painful to watch this articulate man struggle for words . . . I know I must stay positive—it's so hard."

And on: "We were so delighted to see Jack sitting up, smiling and alert when we arrived at 1:30. He was talking in sentences, lucid and aware . . . He had a spinal tap at 2 a.m. and again in the mid-morning . . . When the pressure is not on his brain from excess fluid, he is so much better.

"I am encouraged—just hearing him talk normally makes me believe that some day this will be behind us."

Thanksgiving

Thursday, November 22

ELLEN WRITES OF DINNER with family and friends, "When we have dinner, I tearfully thank God that we're all together and that Jack is getting better . . . There is much laughter and good fun." Still, "I miss Jack being there . . . but we must continue to believe that he'll be back here again soon."

The day after Thanksgiving, Jack headed down again. This seems the cruelest trick. Each moment she dares to hope that the worst has passed simply becomes prelude to another setback. Dan Hanley made his first appearance in Ellen's journal that day, November 23, having just returned from a medical conference. Hanley thinks the problem may lie in several small blood vessels rather than one large one. Jack's pattern doesn't fit their expectations, based on other patients' behavior, but that is no cause for alarm. Hanley is encouraging. The infection is slowing.

And so ended the "pattern establishing" days of Jack Apple's story in Ellen Apple's journal, as though it had all been timed deliberately, themes set forth that would repeat over months in variation. Yet no one made anything happen as it did, and no one will make the pattern play on or determine the outcome. Everyone will try to fix the outcome—meaning they will do their best to make it good.

AFTER HANLEY'S ENCOURAGEMENT, Ellen was hopeful enough that she became angry when a nurse said she believed Jack would probably always have major word-finding problems. "No, I will not listen to these negative thoughts," she wrote. "He is going to get better."

Down days: Hanley asks Jack if he knows where he is. Is this a hospital or a supermarket? "Jack says 'Supermarket,' probably repeating the last word he heard." Jack identifies his daughter and daughter-in-law correctly, but not Ellen or their son. "When Dr. Hanley asks Doug's relationship to him, he mumbles, 'Sister.' "

Up days: "The MRI this morning showed no permanent brain damage, only some irritation where the drain had been in his head. *This is good news.*"

Finally the up days were stringing together. Hanley said Jack should be home in two weeks—that would be mid-December—and wrote on his disability form that he would be able to return to work March 1, 1991.

Then into a new labyrinth.

Christmas week. On the day Dan Hanley said Jack's liver was failing, he already had a plunging red-cell count that was potentially starving his whole body for oxygen, and a fever of 102, and blood sugar raging out of control. Hanley thought hepatitis caused the new problem. Jack's voice was thin and reedy. Ellen summarized Christmas: "the worst day he's had." Now, two days later: "Is this the final blow? It starts to snow." And it snowed on, dazzling and ever more opaque, as friends drove her home. The weeks before had been an unreal patchwork of light and dark, her journal repeating comments like, "After yesterday's miracle, we are discouraged." Jack had fallen out of bed several times, and both Hanley and the nurse he was closest to had urged Ellen to hire a night-duty attendant, which she had done.

The permanent shunt put in to replace the original catheter drain stopped working properly and was revised. Jack went from normally conversational on some days, when Ellen would write of what great buddies he and Hanley had become, to morose and uncommunicative, to rambling incoherently. Even Hanley seemed to be preparing her for the worst. We are probably at Square 2 or 3, he had said, and it may be a long way to Square 4, let alone 10. "He intimates that Jack may never . . . be able to make new memories," she wrote.

He rebounds miraculously when their children are there.

Then, "When I arrive home, I listen to messages. The last is from Jack. He insists that I come and get him, as he is being held prisoner in a third-rate prison."

Twelve hours later: "This is the best day yet."

Why the wild swings, usually from morning (high) to night (low)? John Ulatowski, an attending neurointensivist, calls it "sundowning" and lays it to pressure in Jack's brain still not being regulated properly—but that is a solvable problem, he encourages her.

Up: "Six weeks today! Jack looks well and is very coherent."

Down: "Not a good day . . . In six weeks he has gone from a vigorous, productive person to a frail old man."

More bad weather. A few days before New Year's it began to snow just before Ellen and her friends left Johns Hopkins. As they drove for home, the snowstorm increased and traffic slowed as cars skidded. By the time they reached Northern Parkway, halfway home, the combination of snow and abandoned vehicles was so bad they decided to stop and have dinner. She called the hospital and was told Jack's night attendant could not make it to work in the storm. After dinner, Ellen asked her friends to take her back to Johns Hopkins. They stayed in the waiting room as she passed the night at Jack's bedside.

Overnight he sank. Soon Hanley was there and ordered Jack's return to the NICU. He introduced Ellen to Michael Diringer, who would manage his case.

The year closes, another opens: "Agonizing . . . No change . . . Breathing somewhat better . . . Kidneys functioning at 10 percent . . . Kidney and liver worse . . .

"I tell Dr. Hanley I am concerned about recovery. He assures me that he feels recovery is possible and will tell me when and if he feels it is not."

Then, after a horrible, rainy night, "Jack awake and responsive today." The next day he is agitated and out of control. "He is wild and I cannot stand to watch his agony."

Two days later, yet another setback, reported to her by NICU nurse Kathy Murphy. "I tell Kathy that I don't want his agony continued," Ellen writes.

"She says, 'Do you mean that if he arrests, you don't want us to resuscitate him?'

"I reply, 'I must talk this over with my children.'"

Hanley still believes Jack can get better. "I say I want him to be left a human being not a vegetable," she writes. "He agrees. He will tell me when he feels it is no longer possible." Hanley urges a family meeting to discuss their various options as the days would unfold. And he gives her this final reassurance: "He will make life-threatening decisions even if I am not there for agreement." He promises resolution. He cannot promise it will be a happy one.

When Hanley feels Jack can no longer emerge a viable person, he will stop aggressive procedures. The next week will be critical. "If he does not start to get better," Ellen writes of Hanley's counsel, "then we may need to have further thoughts about continuing treatment . . .

"Earlier . . . Jack was trying to tell us something we couldn't understand. I leaned down close and he tried to kiss me through the mask. I wish I could just hold him and comfort and calm him. He doesn't deserve this agony."

The Gulf War begins. Jack remembers the country is at war with Iraq but has no idea who or where he is.

January 25. "When I arrive about noon Jack is in a chair playing with his nightgown and will not look at us or talk to us. He reminds me of a mental patient in an institution. I am distraught and pour out all my frustrations to Dr. [Laurel] Moore, telling her I feel betrayed by the doctors who kept telling me he would be all right and could still have a quality life. What I'm seeing now is certainly not quality and doesn't resemble Jack in any way . . .

"I also feel guilt because Jack and I had promised each other we would not allow this to happen. Neither of us want to be kept alive without life."

Resolution.

There are 17 journal entries between January 25 and February 13, 1991, but they offer no transition, disclosing no pattern other than that of a sine wave, rolling between positive and negative extremes. This entry, which looks like fifty percent of the rest, will prove different:

February 13: "It is a good day. He does not get off track at all. They say his speech is very good, and he probably will not need much therapy. He is getting stronger."

What is different? This good day is not followed by a setback. This Wednesday, 14 weeks after Ellen Apple frantically negotiated the maze of construction to reach Johns Hopkins, reveals the end of the hospital road, glimmering ahead. But it is identifiable only in retrospect. Ellen's hopeful, even joyous entries could be paired with others in the past, but each of those was followed by downturn, even disaster. Now there would be only clear sailing, as though foreordained.

February 14: "Valentine's Day! Can you believe he has a card and presents for me?" Daughter Linda bought the presents for him to give. "But the card is written by Jack and expresses so much love. Of course, I cry. He is so aware today, we discuss the car, finances, and the future."

February 16: "He asks to see the diary I've kept since day one . . . He remembers nothing of what happened to him, and can't believe what he is reading. He asks some questions and just keeps saying, 'I never knew I was so sick.'" People from the NICU are amazed at his recovery. "They call him a miracle. And to me he is."

February 17: Visiting the NICU, he looks at the pictures of the nurses he read about in Ellen's diary. "We see Dr. Diringer and he, too, is thrilled to see Jack up and walking." Jack calls all his friends, who are ecstatic.

February 19: "The chest X ray is fine and his swallowing test not perfect but OK. Bernadette [Jack's favorite nurse] says goodbye and the three of us have a very emotional moment—all crying . . . This is the final entry . . . "

January 4, 2001

B A L T I M O R E   L I E S   U N D E R   six inches of snow, squished up into hillocks and depressed into watery troughs in the streets, so walking is at its most difficult, even if your balance is perfect. Still, when Dan Hanley suggests getting lunch in one of the hospital cafeterias, Jack Apple persuades him to head across the street to one that's much better. Apple also takes credit for pointing Hanley to the best Jewish delis in this end of Baltimore, which the corned-beef-loving Hanley had never found on his own. Jack and Ellen, Dan and wife Christine have met regularly for dinner over more than a decade, so their talk is more between friends than doctor and patient, but Jack is still a prime example for Dr. Hanley about what can be done against *nihil*.

Jack returned to work after months of rehabilitation. If parts of his brain were permanently damaged, which is not known, other parts adapted and restored him. Only the tiny hairs in his inner ears remain damaged. He wears a hearing aid, and after one disastrous attempt to ride his bicycle again gave up on that. His balance is still sometimes off, he says.

In all but those ways, Jack's brain has come back all the way. But is it the same collection of neurons, precisely? Or have new cells linked into new networks, providing *the same person* with new ways to apprehend and relate the world? The brain, after all, is the great shapeshifter. The world imprints it, because it evolved to lie open to imprinting by the world. A hand imprints wet clay, in three dimensions. World imprints brain in manifold. Plastic is the term: Bend it this way, it retains the bend; now add a new kink, and that remains, too. A metaphor for learning.

Why did Hanley believe Jack Apple could pull through?

Intracerebral pressure was the first clue. "With Jack, I knew that, first, his ICP was high but not that high, and second, from the scans, there had not been a lot of brain damage. I had to keep him going long enough to get the blood out. I thought in a month it all might resolve."

And then a remarkable comment: "I knew I could keep anybody alive for one month."

Still, the question that nagged at those treating the deadly consequences of such strokes was, Couldn't they find a way to get rid of the clots faster? The complications of these hemorrhages all followed from blood-clotted cerebrospinal fluid channels in those ventricular cisterns, causing them to swell, and from dangerous blood breakdown products damaging the ventricles and brain tissue, leading to edema and hydrocephalus.

Answer: Yes, they could.

As winter wears into summer, Hanley pushes deeper into a major study for which he is co–principal investigator with Hopkins neuro-surgeon Neal Naff. It goes by a daunting title that can be shortened to IVH Thrombolysis. The large multicenter trial aims to learn whether the clot-busting drug TPA, which has had great success in saving victims of heart attacks and ischemic strokes, is also effective in breaking up the clots that kill more than 70 percent of those who initially survive intraventricular hemorrhages. The key to their long-term, slow developing study is that TPA—tissue plasminogen activator in the long form—must not induce new hemorrhages. But how can anyone assure that?

The idea of injecting a clot-dissolving, hence blood-thinning, drug into the ventricles of someone whose brain has been bleeding is entirely counterintuitive. That's why the FDA required, in approving the drug for heart attacks and ischemic strokes, that the label warn it was not to be used by anyone who has had a hemorrhage, Hanley notes. And that's why it took many years for investigators to get to this large clinical trial on a drug in use for 20 years.

By July, 2001, the evidence was clearly pointing to TPA as a life saver. The patient enrollment was still too small to talk in percentages, but it was clear that the number of TPA-dosed patients surviving their hemorrhages and recovering was well beyond the predicted survival rate, which was based on past evidence. The key to success, researchers believe, is to inject a small dose of the drug directly into the ventricles, where the clots are, rather than giving it systemically, where it would affect all the blood vessels. They do not admit patients into the trial who have had bleeding aneurysms, because those are likely to rebleed, and there are other disqualifiers. In other words, they have identified a subset of patients amenable to treatment. If all goes as Hanley believes it will, some years down the road TPA will routinely be given to some victims of intraventricular stroke.

I T W O U L D B E G O O D right now on this clear, breezy summer day for the medical corps of Johns Hopkins to have a diagnostic tool to foresee onrushing events as they, like the rhythms of the brain, line up into cataclysm. Instead, most get the bad news on the evening news, as the rest of the world does, or they read it tomorrow morning, July 20, in the *Baltimore Sun:*

> Seven weeks after the death of a young woman in an asthma study, the federal government suspended human medical experiments at the Johns Hopkins University yesterday because of what regulators characterized as widespread lapses in safety procedures.

Dead in the water: 2,400 human experiments involving 15,000 patients and volunteers. But that was only the beginning. The $419 million Johns Hopkins received in federal funds this year was by far more than that going to any other university or institute, and $255 million of that is to conduct research on people. How many multicenter clinical trials now hung frozen? Hard to say, but what stopped here stopped at most of the other centers as well, for four days, until the university was allowed to begin, however cautiously.

Trina Cunningham, last seen in yellow OR gown bearing informed consent papers, has a board on her office wall tracking in code some of what is now frozen: IHAST2, ALSIUS, WASID.

To those add IVH Thrombolysis. Naff and Hanley's multicenter trial with TPA is in limbo. Visit Columbia and researchers talk about their participation as one of those multicenters being halted while everything gets sorted out. Romer Geocadin's investigation into cardiac arrest stops.

As the government lifts restrictions over coming days and weeks, trials with direct benefit to patients are allowed to resume first. That means the TPA intraventricular hemorrhage and other studies resume, at a much slower pace as new regulations are put in place, learned and followed. Studies in the pilot stage, which are not at the point of demonstrating direct patient benefit, are delayed far longer, so it is months before Geocadin gets his cardiac arrest study back on track.

IN HIS OFFICE, Edward Miller, former head of anesthesia and critical care medicine, now dean of medicine and CEO of Johns Hopkins, has cooled since his angry reply to the federal Office of Human Research Protections. Cooled, but not changed his view that the shutdown was botched, an overreaction to a genuine tragedy that came weeks after the hospital itself had taken the appropriate action.

What the feds should have done was conducted a "focused shutdown" that would have suspended studies on volunteers, not clinical trials on sick patients, many of whom were in desperate need of the experimental therapies they were getting.

Miller is in his office next to the dome, where he delivered his angry rebuttal to the research office in a press conference. The office is spacious, needing its large conference table, chairs, and couches for less formal discussions.

Miller still believes OHRP "did not understand the magnitude of research here and the number of patients affected.

"All leukemic children are on protocols. Every child. The reason is, we still don't know what's the best protocol in each case." That is now a familiar theme: once you know a treatment works best, you must end the trial. Until then, you must continue, because hunches don't work; you really don't know what's best.

"Patients were on a vaccine for pancreatic cancer. There were drug addiction and weight loss programs that stopped." And the stoppage hit all the partnering medical centers.

But let's pause a moment. What happened was the unthinkable in medical research, and everyone encountered has been left somber by it.

Consider: A 24-year-old woman named Ellen Roche, who loves horses and owns her own, who has just bought a home, volunteers to help investigators try to learn what goes wrong in the lungs of asthma sufferers when they get hit by the sort of minor irritations that the rest of us fend off without knowing it. She is given an inhalation of the drug hexamethonium, which is intended to give her and the other healthy volunteers precisely that challenge, a minor irritation. But she develops a bad cough quickly, and overnight her breathing gets worse. She is hospitalized at Bayview, where she works, and the best doctors work to save her. But nothing stops the ravages of this drug on her, and it ravages her alone. She dies in a few weeks, her lungs destroyed, the entire armamentarium of modern medicine powerless to save her.

A thousand questions sprang to mind over succeeding weeks, but clearly the most important question for the future is, Will all the new requirements prevent a recurrence?

Miller answers that question by offering a different scenario of the events leading up to the tragedy, because it is in the scenario that he sees the real error having been made. One of the volunteers given the drug *before* Roche also developed a cough, and she was properly removed from the trial.

"When the first patient coughed, had symptoms, that should have ended it—right there, that's when the trial should have been suspended," Miller says. "Yet patients were still enrolled. That's the one place we can look and say that [researcher Dr. Alkis Togias] should have rethought the thing.

"Togias made a clinical judgment. We never thought [the error] was done in a cavalier manner. If he had reported the first patient's cough and he'd changed his procedure as a result, and *then* someone had died, we would have done everything possible to prevent it."

Others within medicine were far harsher. Adil E. Shamoo, a University of Maryland biochemist who is often critical of human experimentation, noted that hexamethonium had previously been shown to cause lung problems—it was unusual for it do so, perhaps, *but it had happened.*

Shamoo, editor of the journal *Accountability in Research,* told the *Baltimore Sun,* "This is not a medication. This is a very toxic chemical. The interest of scientists should never supersede the interest of patients."

What had been interrupted eventually resumed. The clinical trials— Hanley's intraventricular hemorrhage protocol, Geocadin's efforts to discriminate those who survived cardiac arrest from those who did not—all coursed back into the current of analyses that had been flowing right along, like Mirski's on the intensivist-managed NICU. Looked at dead on, all the data streams emerge as a kind of snapshot of the present, like page one of a newspaper or the table of contents of a medical journal.

AS FOR MIRSKI'S PUBLICATIONS, they draw discussion and comment everywhere he goes, as intended. The ICU, he notes, is one of the highest-cost units in the entire hospital. He has found increasing evidence that his structure will cut those costs by improving patient outcome. Now, the *Journal of the American Medical Association* has published several reports leading large companies to demand management of ICUs by intensivists.

There is just one problem: some hospitals demand that "intensivist" mean board-certified specialists in critical-care medicine, if not in internal medicine, anesthesia, or one of the other specialties that lack neuroscience training, but do focus on the rest of the patient. Such a demand would squeeze out the neurologists from their own subspecialty. Mirski has just been on the phone with Tom Bleck, one of the earliest pioneers and the neurointensivist at the University of Virginia. Bleck has been in conversations with the Society of Critical Care Medicine and the American Academy of Neurology in an attempt to solve the problem. The long way around would be for neurointensivists to win their own board certification, under the neurology academy. But all they need is for hospitals—and the large insurance payers—to demand only that neurocritical care units be run by doctors with subspecialty training in any area of critical care. Bleck is in a strong position because he is also board certified in critical care, as Mirski is in anesthesia.

At Columbia, Stephan Mayer puts the finishing touches on the approach he and a handful of others have been working on for months:

incorporating the Society for Neurocritical Care in New York. The list of co-incorporators is impressive, including Wade Smith and Claude Hemphill of the University of California at San Francisco, who conduct a large portion of the fellowship program focused on neurotrauma; Jeffrey Frank of the University of Chicago, and Gene Sung of the University of Southern California.

They are heavyweights from major units in this new field, but will they succeed in getting their training programs accepted into the world of medical specialties, not only by their colleagues but by such powerful groups as Leapfrog, the payers of health insurance? Will their first meeting be a convention of the converted, leaving the organization without influence? The final answer to the big question could take the better part of a decade to resolve. But even that second, smaller question would require a journey of nearly two years to answer.

CHAPTER 11

"Catherine Is Dying"

Johns Hopkins Hospital
February 20, 2002

Before Stephan Mayer turned Antonia Gonzalez's respirator off that July day, her family had gathered in total silence just beyond her bed on the eighth floor of Columbia's New York Presbyterian Hospital. The atmosphere is as somber here today. It's impossible not to reflect back, then forward, then back again.

Passing by Catherine Demarest's room, everyone's gaze is drawn to the young couple sitting by her bed. Their body language, their posture, pulls at you. And even if you hadn't seen Catherine's chart, the vibrant blonde hair poking above the swath of bandages suggests she's young. The chart says she is 29.

Both man and woman, about the same age, are taking what they've heard pretty hard, she visibly more so than he. Brother and sister? Could be, but no. Brian Johnson is Catherine's husband, Chris Demarest her sister.

Before ushering them into her room, a nurse had prepared them for what to expect: no movement, no recognition, eyes closed. A tube in her mouth to help her breathe. A tube surgically placed in her head for pressure control. MVA—motor vehicle accident. "She can't talk to you, but feel free to talk to her. There are monitors for her heart – and other monitors. Don't let them bother you."

"She looks asleep," Chris says tearfully.

Chere Chase has come in. "Let me get you some tissues," she says, touching Chris on the shoulder.

"They did get the blood clot out," Brian says, half hopeful statement, half question.

"They did," Chase says. "One of our biggest concerns now, though, is pressure on her brain. The surgery was successful. As the brain tries to heal itself, it often swells, and that can cause damage." Pause. "Right now, we don't know how reversible her injuries might be. Some of her injuries could lead to permanent deficits."

"You mean," Chris Demarest says, voice breaking, "she could be in a wheelchair or something?"

"We don't know yet."

"She's a strong woman," Chris shoots back. "She's very healthy. She's stubborn. She's a fighter."

"Please understand," Chase says, leaning close, looking her straight in the eyes. "We're worried she may not make it through the day. We're hopeful she'll respond."

"Oh, she will!" Chris says. "She can't die. She can't die."

Brian, who looks to be in his early thirties, rarely speaks, except to ask for explanation of something he didn't follow, then wants facts. Otherwise he sits, elbows on knees, neck slumped between shoulders, staring ahead.

Evening.

"There are parts of her brain not injured. But if we can't control the pressure, that could damage the healthy parts. Our unit involves both neurosurgeons and critical-care doctors. We're using medical therapy now, but if we need to, we can call on the neurosurgeons."

Chris: "She's still under anesthesia, right? She *can't* wake up."

Chase: "Her unconsciousness is more related to her brain injury, and her brain pressure. We hope as we decrease the pressure, we'll see her wake up more."

A nurse says to Brian, "Would you like us to call someone? We have chaplains here."

Chris jumps in: "She doesn't need last rites or anything!" More challenge than question.

But Brian gets the idea. "Her folks are very old and frail. They're out of state. They couldn't get here if they wanted to."

Chase: "I wish I could give you better news. It concerns me that this long after surgery we're not seeing more response."

Brian: "She's not conscious at all?"

Chase: "I would describe her as in a deep state of coma. I hope we can get control over this pressure and that she'll be able to recover from this."

Morning.

The chaplain has been here off and on, now sits quietly between Brian and Chris. "Dr. Chase will be here soon," she says. "I saw her in the hallway." As Chase comes in, husband and sister jump to their feet, Chris Demarest wringing her hands as she talks. First, they had gotten an early morning phone call saying Catherine had gotten worse rather than better, then came the news when they arrived that the doctors had found *no sign* of brain activity.

It takes only a few moments for Brian Johnson to come to the point: "We thought the worst, " he says. "But she doesn't look different. She doesn't look worse."

And a brief moment to respond: "There is *no* normal function of her brain," Chase says. "And the injury to her brain is so severe she is no longer able to breathe on her own. We're concerned her brain injuries may lead to her passing away."

"No, no, no!" Chris pleads. "People are in comas for months, for years and they come out of comas."

Chase, the chaplain and the nurses have all been assiduously laying the groundwork for this, trying to reduce the shock, from the moment yesterday Chase had warned, "we're worried she may not make it through the day." But the determined brushback of the unthinkable is as much hope as denial, though the denial is powerfully evident. Miracles *do* happen. We've read about them in books and seen them on TV. Some witness them firsthand, others have lived them.

Chase says in her solid, steady voice, "Unfortunately, her coma is to the point that she cannot be taken off life support."

"Never?"

"No."

"She's dead?" Brian says in a level voice. "She can't be gone!"

"I wish I had better news. Her trauma is so severe that I don't believe she'll be able to sustain life without —"

Chris hurries out of the room, Brian slowly follows, and soon the conversation resumes in the family waiting room, at first just among the three of them.

Chase: "The pressure in her brain is too severe for her to survive."

Chris: "What are you going to do to help her?"

Brian leans toward Chase. "She's still fighting, right?"

Chase slowly, firmly shakes her head. "The pressure has been too great."

Brian: "Is there any possibility at all she'll get better?"

"No," Chase says simply. "I wish I could say otherwise, but the pressure on her brain was too severe." First use of the past tense.

Chris breaks into sobs.

Chase: "I wish I could offer better. There is nothing we can do, surgically or medically. If over the next hours there is no change, that means she has died. Both the nurses' team and the doctors' team did everything we could. Her injuries were too severe for her to survive."

Chaplain: "Is there someone we need to call for you? Friends, to let them know she's dying?"

"They've moved," Brian says. "I don't think they're going to come."

Nurse: "Would you like to go back to her room, to be with her?"

Chris stares at her a few moments, nods, then she and Brian head back to see Catherine one last time, ending now as they began the morning before. It closes as a triptych, the right and the left morning panels focusing on the middle: Sometime during the night, Catherine died.

"YOU NOTICE HOW Chris the sister gets all the attention?" Mike Williams asks, commenting on the long performance the group gathered around the television monitor has just witnessed. It has been a performance, but in more important ways, a reenactment. "She shows her emotions, her heart is on her sleeve, and everyone wants to comfort her. But look over there at poor old Brian."

And there, on the monitor, Brian "men-don't-show-pain" sits slumped by the hospital bed like stone, until the chaplain moves to his side and puts her arm around his shoulders—fairly early in the four-hour run of this drama. Williams's conversation takes place in a control room next to a stage, and what has been going on with Brian, Chris, a dummy, and a very real, very involved Dr. Chere Chase, three nurses and a chaplain is as serious as death to everyone here, but this dying and its end were improvised to help them deal with the real ones.

Onlookers who know exactly what is going on fight back tears they would never allow themselves to show in the NICU, because this is no skit. It's a replay of a thousand days of their professional lives, and the separate "acts" of the event are broken by critical, often deeply felt commentary on how the medical professionals reacted to what was thrown at them without warning.

Tom Wyatt as Brian Johnson and Mary Donovan as Chris Demarest are professional actors, trained not only as straight dramatic actors but in improv, further trained through conferences with Mike Williams and other physicians and nurses, in the dynamics of family-medical interactions, as they are lived every day. Their job, carried out with realistic gusto, is to simply react as they believe they would – as family members confronted with unthinkable events, in an effort to deal with the real ones. What makes this doctor's response assuage a distraught family, and this other's response, that appears no different, upset them and eventually split them into opposing camps? In other words, this is a kind of laboratory experiment. It's run under controls and meeting truth-tests too rough for scientific validity, but it aims to get at things science so far can't reach. The "human heart," for example.

The scenes enacted are uncomfortably real for most of the participants, each moment, gesture, and distraught question twisted into the fabric of so many working days. All their patients are critically ill. Most get well, but many die.

Ski Lower had pointed out that families often prod NICU nurses for information, thinking they'll get a simpler answer with fewer confusing qualifications, than they'd get from doctors. But if the truth is that "your husband doesn't stand a prayer," what do you say?

Lower: "I tell them, 'We will do everything within our power to pull him through, but in my experience, most patients with this severity of this type of illness do not survive.' I may lead up to it, or I may put it that simply. But if that's the truth, that's what I want them to hear."

ANTONIA GONZALEZ. Noon. A nurse is trying to track down Dr. Mayer, who is four floors down from Columbia's NICU giving a Department of Medicine grand rounds on terminal extubation. She wants to tell him Antonia's family is ready. They have talked over the case and they've discussed the wishes of their daughter, sister, aunt. They're ready for the doctor to remove her tube one last time—to terminally extubate her—and turn off her ventilator. As Mayer talks one of his several pagers goes off, the one that means 'drop everything.' He excuses himself to the physicians and students in the audience, steps to the side of the dais, and phones upstairs. The resident suggests that someone else do the extubation. "No," Mayer says. "I promised. I'm on my way up."

"Sorry," he tells the group, "I won't have time for Q and A."

Back in his speedwalk, slide carousel tucked under his arm, he heads for Antonia and her family. Exiting the elevator, he passes the broad window whose view seems a blue-green abstract, the gunmetal and rust of the Palisades across the river streaked with leafy green white dots of sails beneath on the river. Hurries through the unit's double doors, arrives at Antonia's bed. The assemblage is unmistakable. Half a dozen family members cluster around a tall man in Roman collar. *"El señor es mi pastor,"* he says, beginning the Twenty-third Psalm.

There are two components of consciousness, Mayer had said to his rounding team at Michael Sanders's bed. *Wakefulness and mental activity. Is the
light on in there? That's wakefulness, pure brain stem, fairly easy to determine.
But is anybody home? That's much harder to decide.*

When Mayer had pinched Sanders, he took the eye saccade shot straight
at him—anger?—as a sign that indeed someone was home. Confused,
dim, not all there, but someone on his way back. The next day new reactions continued to prove him right. Not so with Antonia. The light was
on, but there was nothing more. She had said to her family, Don't leave me
like that. Carlos Gonzalez, Antonia's brother, served the most critical function in this set piece: family spokesman.

This is where it can get very sticky in some circumstances. Mike
Williams said, "When I talk to families and I ask important questions, I
always try to pick up on whether everyone's eyes tend to go toward one
person to provide the answers. It's good if there is such a person, because
you can also get disagreement, confusion, cross-purposes, people with
entirely different understandings of what's going on and what should
happen—none of them wrong."

In Antonia's case, her brother rather than her mother, who is also
right at her side, has been designated next of kin. He is also the only family member fluent in English. What can be a drawback in some circumstances is a boon in these, because in translating Carlos also explains what
he has been told.

The responsive *amen* concluding the psalm, eliding to Mayer's explanation of what he will do, makes his actions seem part of the last
rites. He walks to Antonia's side and listens to the respirator for a moment. Her breathing is *apneustic,* a dense small word meaning she in-
hales with a stutter, because the automatic nerve signals from her brain
stem are not working as they should; they may be shutting down. He

turns off the ventilator, and, as expected, she begins to breathe in the same halting way on her own. Now he quickly withdraws from Antonia's throat the metal tube that kept her airway open and carried the line for heavily oxygenated air. He studies the charts. The nurse records the readings from the many monitors: blood pressure, blood oxygen and carbon dioxide, red cell count. Mayer reads off the time of day. Thus begins the countdown that will continue long after Mayer leaves for the day, though he will return frequently. The family stays with her, some with heads bowed, others talking or silently weeping.

What is the function of the four-hour interactive discourse toward Catherine's death at Johns Hopkins—a ritual now spreading to other medical centers? One doctor, one resident, one nurse hardly ever follows a case like Antonia's from beginning to end. They find themselves in midshift forced to jump into a role whose first scenes were carried out by others. Patients who are so near death they seem one missed breath away sometimes live for days, or simply go into that end stage called persistent vegetative. The light remains on, the ventilator remains on, but no one ever returns. Such patients are taken to nursing homes, often by way of the hospital section called Intermediate Care Unit, where many of the patients linger in this twilight zone. Eventually, they fail the brain tests and are pronounced dead, years after they last took part in the world.

Sometime during the early hours of the morning after Mayer extubated her, Antonia Gonzalez died. Here is how it was known.

The on-call resident was wakened in the call room by a page from the nurse on Antonia's floor. He returned the page from the phone by his bed. Antonia had stopped breathing. He hurried up to her unit. The light was out.

First he—the junior resident—called the senior resident, who is allowed to take call from home, and they reviewed how to perform the brain stem test. The resident brushed a tissue against the corneas of Antonia's open eyes. Nothing. The eyes are the only external organs whose touch receptors are only for pain. That is, there is nothing that is supposed to feel good brushing against your eyes. If the eyes do not reflexively close on being touched, that is a fatal sign. Antonia had lost both her cough and gag reflexes, two other lower brain-stem reflexes. Either of these can be lost to a small brain stem stroke that spares other vital structures. That's why each test, like each step of the neurological exam, is cumulative and intended to reflect its own special brain function. Now there is one test left. The principal brain stem reflexes for the ear and the eye are adjacent to one another. If you pour cold water into a person's left ear canal, both eyes should look to the right, away from the "insult." If you pour in warm water, the eyes should look left, toward the pleasant sensation. In Antonia's case, there was nothing.

Since she was already off the respirator, there was nothing more to be done. Death was confirmed at that moment. It was approximately 15 hours after Mayer had performed the terminal extubation and turned off the ventilator.

SOME TRAINING ENACTS scenarios that have never happened, as preparation for the first time, such as those for biowarfare. "Catherine Is Dying" represents art distilling reality, the events that normally cover many hours and that can stretch over months compressed into a day of engagement and discussion.

Dozens of times a year in the Neuro ICU such scenes with families are repeated in variations as complex as people, as families. Multiply that for medical, surgical, pediatric ICUs. Multiply that by the number of units on the floor, where patients are not critical but can become so and die within minutes. And multiply that by the number of vanguard hospitals treating the sickest patients, and factor in those small community hospitals where patients also lapse into coma and die. More and more, thanks to the technological innovations of the operating room and emergency room now in the hands of intensivists, death comes by decisions like these, rather than a blunt "lights out."

M ORNING ROUNDS STILL BEGIN at 8 at Johns Hopkins. Major changes are coming, and though they can't be foreseen at this point, everyone on the NICU team is already feeling the pressure of increased responsibilities. Bayview is well under way, successfully, and that will mean increased demand for the intensivists' services there. The new NICU here is half open, but so far the number of intensive care beds hasn't increased; some old beds have simply been replaced with new. Not that you'd notice on morning rounds. The focus is always on what's tracking and beeping on the color monitor over the patient, the readouts from the many leads plugging in data from the lungs, heart, and blood. For patients whose intracranial pressure is being monitored via a bolt inserted in the top of the skull, those data add their own lines on the screen. Otherwise, if your attention wanders, you notice that rooms along one side of the unit are new, their colors soft and muted, yet somehow the net effect brighter than in the old.

Mike Williams is attending this week, soon to be followed by Marek Mirski, who is now in the operating room. Room 731, untouched by the remodelers so far, is the team's first stop. The new drill begins as always here, with the patient's incoming nurse reading the report passed along by the overnight nurse.

Obi Okoye was Rita Serianni's nurse on the eve of her transfer from the intensive care unit to a rehabilitation facility where, with care and luck, she would continue the recovery that had so far been promising. On

July 24, Okoye said in the discharge report that the immediate neurological treatment goal was to optimize cerebral perfusion. *The skull must make room for three things, blood, CSF and brain itself,* Mirski had said in teaching rounds. Cerebral perfusion—CPP—indicates the pressure within brain tissue itself.

The nurses have to be as well-versed in these dynamics as the doctors, and Okoye has reached the top nursing rank, Nurse Clinician III. Leaving her native Anambra Province in eastern Nigeria in 1986, she came to Johns Hopkins in 1993, with a bachelor of science in nursing and a few years experience as a nurse in medicine. Years of experience, classes, and exams had led her through the nurse-clinician levels to this third.

Continuing Serianni's exit report: "Blood pressure and sodium goals have been met," Okoye said. "No seizures"—a very good sign. Along with her sodium goal came the information that Serianni was being given 2 percent salt water solution at 200 cc's per hour to maintain that balance because she was still at risk for hydrocephalus—which she had had days ago, but it was clearing up. She is being given the antiseizure medication Kepra as a preventative, because she is still at risk for seizure as well. Fortunately, her vasospasm is also clearing up. She appears past the major danger point of having a cerebral arteries clamp down, bringing on a stroke.

The rest of the neuro exam can be summed up quickly in Stephan Mayer's phrase: the lights are on. Now on to other important issues. How much is she aware of what is going on around her? "She is flexing at best," Okoye read. That meant Rita Serianni was not alert enough to dart an angry glance at Williams if he pinched her arm or to yank her hand away if he pressed a car key into a fingernail base. Her upper, hemispheric brain would have to coordinate those commands. Instead, her upper brain stem brought on the pain reflex of pulling back extremities, toward the body center, when pain struck. This was a better stage of recovery than extending in response to pain – sticking out arms and stretching feet – the reflex of the still-more primitive lower brain stem.

IS SHE HOME YET? Someone is stirring, that's clear. When Phil and the girls come in, every day without fail, Rita rouses slightly. When they hold her hand, she often inclines her head toward them, sometimes even smiles to that gesture or the sound of their voices, which could be a sign that the neurons of the upper brain are resuming their coordinated dance that somehow emerges as personhood.

Yesterday she had a PEG line inserted, a tube that would provide permanent nutrition directly into her stomach rather than intravenously. And she was given a tracheotomy so she could breathe without the metal tube extending from her mouth down into her throat. That will not only reduce the risk of infection but will allow her more freedom to respond orally when asked questions as she recovers.

Phil and their daughters work to bring her around, and Rita responds, gains ground through August. Her birthday is September 2, and they buy presents and prepare a birthday party for her bedside. Phil is troubled that nearly two months after surgery she is not awake and alert, but she does seem to be slowly responding to them, and many different outcomes would be better than nothing.

A phone call in the middle of the night rarely brings good news. The voice on September 2 told him Rita had just died. An onset of pneumonia had killed her, that quickly. That was it. It was over.

WITH TIME PASSING, "it gets better," Serianni said over coffee the next March 3. "But it never gets good."

Rita's death after the agonizing months of ups and downs hit them all terribly hard, and perhaps not surprisingly was hardest on Natalie,

Suzanne, and Monica. They had lingered at home, unbelieving at first, having a hard time getting back to their separate lives.

Phil had gone back to work almost immediately, but he was glad they had all made the decision to get professional counseling, to help them through. To make life better even if, for him, it was a dicey proposition whether it would get good again. He runs three days a week and works out in the gym, and looks it. He stays trim. He does not want to be too quick to say that what happened was for the worst. It might have been God's gift.

"Rita had always said she would not want to live in a wheelchair," Serianni says. "It's been an awful year. Her sister died last January, even younger than Rita. When I think of it that way, from what the doctors told me, she might have always been in a wheelchair. Or even worse off. And she wouldn't have wanted that. Maybe God was right." What's plain is that, so far, it doesn't feel right.

TAMMY BRASHER STRUGGLED, determined to live out her brave words, but it sure wasn't easy. On August 8, a few weeks after her discharge, Joe Rose had to take Tammy back to the hospital. Infection had plagued her since a few months after her first surgery, at a community hospital near where they lived. Olivi had been worried about it in July, cleared it the best he could, and attempted to repair the damaged membranes covering and protecting the brain after he'd placed her Gliadel wafer. Now when Olivi looked, he could see that the tumor was not the major problem; it was infection. The infection had to be controlled quickly, because it was causing swelling. By the end of summer, Tammy was wheelchair bound. But she and the children were now living with Joe and his mother, JoAnn, in their home in north Baltimore. They would marry as soon as Tammy was able, and Joe would adopt Krystal and Michael, who had just celebrated their tenth and ninth birthdays. She told Joe and the kids she would be out of the wheelchair in no time.

At the very end of September, Tammy returned for yet more neurosurgery, this time so Olivi could place a shunt to drain the edema from the infection. The morning after, October 1, Joe got a call at work. It was Tammy, bright and alert, telling him how much she loved him, and how good she felt with the pressure relieved. Soon she was up and walking. Olivi called the whole staff together to watch and applaud her.

They had to postpone the wedding because the infection came back. No matter; she fought it. Olivi operated to drain the infection and she fought it some more. Through it all, one after another of the Baltimore Ravens squad visited, brought her gifts, cheered her up. The year 2001 became 2002, then winter became spring, summer, fall. Through all the ups and downs, she continued walking, and when she was up, there was always that same spark. She would not give in. They set their wedding date for October 25 and filed adoption papers. But they had to postpone the wedding. Tammy had more brain infection and soon developed a lung infection as well.

On December 22, at 4:21 a.m., she died in Joe's arms at a local hospital. A lung infection was listed as cause of death. At about 4:30 p.m. on Christmas Eve, Tammy's ex, Tim Healey, came to the Roses to take Krystal and Michael to live with him and his wife in Alabama. Joe says they did not want to leave, but Healey got a court order, and they went. The day after Christmas, Tammy Brasher, 32, was buried. Among the mourners Joe counted Alex Olivi. Joe was touched to see the doctor had tears in his eyes.

Lazarus

Johns Hopkins Hospital

April

T HERE ARE SOME weeks when the large new unit is half-empty, and the relatively few patients are all postop and recovering well. Work that's been put off gets done. Diana Greene-Chandos had just changed her research direction, leaving a collaboration with Anish Bhardwaj and joining one with Michel Torbey, whose interests seemed more clinical to her, more directly related to her interests as a bedside doctor. She prayed for one of those slow weeks now, because her son Connor's second birthday was coming up, and she needed a little slack to prepare his party.

Along came the other kind of week. All the patients were terribly sick, or so it seemed. Rounds drew longer and were more frequently interrupted by emergencies. One of the nurses fell ill with mononucleosis, so they had to get a replacement. Did she catch it from a patient? Hard to tell; they were all running ragged and tired—nurses, attendings, fellows.

The research demand at Johns Hopkins was one kind of powerful gravitational pull. The pull of the clinic was entirely different. It was immediate, the demand of patients needing round-the-clock care that matched point for point what all the previous training had been about. For many, they complemented one another. But for both Chere Chase and Diana Greene-Chandos, there was a third force that brought its own compulsion: home. Last July, with so much to be learned anew and the grinding reiteration of residents' rounds, had been stressful to be sure. But her mother had been there for Connor. Soon Diana discovered that leaving to pick up her son was not considered acceptable at this place, not because she stinted on her clinical duties; she never had. But because she was not sacrificing enough for research. She never sensed this from Dr. Mirski. *A real champion of women, of a balanced life,* she often thought. But as often she would reflect on how his wife, Dr. Lenore Nii, had sacrificed her own medical practice to stay home with their daughters.

There are sacrifices you have to make to be at Johns Hopkins. Her son barely recognized her now.

Wednesday she dragged herself home, tired, with a pain in her abdomen that persisted. Nonetheless, she made it through the week. Saturday was quiet, but as though to make up for it, she felt exhausted and listless. The more she pushed, the worse she felt. By the time she got home, she was feverish.

Febrile, a word usually reserved for patients. Her fever soared. She ate some soup but couldn't hold it down. So, just as she might tell a patient *never* to do, she began taking the remainder of a Cipro prescription many months old. It was no help. By Sunday, Dr. Brendan Chandos refused to listen to her insistence that she would be fine and took her with him to St. Agnes Hospital, where she was admitted with a fever of 101 degrees. She had mononucleosis, a viral infection. Making matters worse, her doctors were sure she also had a bacterial infection, but they couldn't grow it out in culture; probably the Cipro had repressed it far enough that it wouldn't show itself.

Sunday night, Chere Chase showed up. As soon as she saw Diana's numbers she grew alarmed. *My God, you're really sick!* They talked a bit, as much as Diana's strength would allow. She dozed. Awakening, there was Chere napping on the next bed, worried that Diana wasn't being watched closely enough. "Chere, you're going to oversleep and miss rounds!" "No," Chere assured her, "I'll wake up in time."

"So there the two of us lay all night," Chase recalled. "Neither of us getting any rest to speak of, me waking up to make sure she was okay, her waking up to make sure I didn't miss rounds." She didn't.

Very slowly, Greene-Chandos began to recover and, as people often do in slowly pulling back from deep, fevered illness, began to think in a long perspective. She was torn. The fellowship and its entailments were her years-old dream, the culmination of her training as a neuroscientist. But she missed her son; she felt he was growing up without her, without knowing her as his mother. Then there was the fact that she and Brendan wanted more children. Over days she felt pulled first one way, then the next. She talked to Brendan, she talked to Chere; yet she came no closer to resolving the contradiction of her demands. She was on the horns of a dilemma, all right, facing two demands that could be neither resolved nor reduced by process of elimination. Then one morning a priest came by, one of the hospital chaplains, asking if she needed anything. She thought for a bit. Yes, she needed some advice.

So she carefully articulated each side of her problem, and she hung in anticipation of his response.

"But you can't leave!" he told her. "You have a calling. You must go on." He had an answer, just as she'd hoped. And in a flash came Diana's epiphany. It was not the answer she had wanted to hear. In choosing someone she unconsciously believed would represent *traditional values,* she was hoping to hear an entirely different answer. Now she knew without doubt what she had been hoping to hear. Sartre could not have laid it out better.

When she returned to the unit a week later, Greene-Chandos told Marek Mirski she had decided to end her fellowship at the one-year point. She was not prepared to simply settle into life as a clinical neurologist, though; she cared too much about the needs of critically ill neuro patients to do that. She would look for a compromise that would allow more time with her family. There was no persuading her otherwise, though Mirski tried. And Chere, determined to push on herself no matter what, was deeply sorry to lose her company as they drew near their second and final year.

Not that all was rosy in Dr. Chase's world. She was strapped for money. Her medical school debts presented mortgage-sized bills every month, and although her grandmother still worked *and* cared for her mother back in Pittsburgh, her grandmother was over 80 now and could not continue forever. Chere began hunting for moonlighting opportunities. By May, she found one. During her off-clinic hours, she began working as an occupational-health intake physician, giving physical exams to people applying for disability, overseeing preemployment drug screening and the like. The Baltimore Metropolitan Transit Authority, with its round-the-clock subway and bus work shifts, was among the clients, so the center was open 24 hours a day. That meant Chase could match her own off-duty schedule. Time-consuming but undemanding compared with her normal duties, it helped balance her budget. She wasn't ahead, but at least she drew even.

The weeks marched on in step, building up—or so it seemed in retrospect—to one hellish week in June.

Greene-Chandos still shared fellow's duties with Chase, and though
she would be gone next month, by then two new junior fellows and a senior fellow returning from leave would swell the ranks of physicians available in the unit. But that new year opening in July seemed to recede as this
week drew on. Five patients would die, but that wasn't the strangest part.

CHRISTINA MANNING was DOA, or at least on arrival she had
met the first of that pair of complex tests that determined her to be brain
dead. She was a young, divorced mother who was now in a homosexual
relationship, and her partner, Anna, was utterly devoted to her and un-
willing to admit she was gone. There was a lot to enable her denial. The
neurointensivists, as always, were maintaining Christina's heartbeat, keeping her blood pressure sky high to drive blood into the unresponsive upper and lower brain. Her brain stem initially began showing slight signs
of life, but not a blip came from any brain structure above it.

Christina had AIDS, and the disease had wracked her kidneys and liver,
which were failing rapidly. It had also left her with endocarditis, an inflammation of the heart that can frequently shoot off small blood clots,
any one of which could be instantly fatal. In this case, those emboli had
traveled to Manning's brain some time ago, producing a series of small
strokes that hospitalized her long before her appearance in the NICU.
Now, Chase and Mike Williams, the attending this week, saw yet another
series of strokes appearing on her CT scans. She also had a high fever.
Now the death knell. Manning appeared to have had a hemorrhagic stroke
that was bleeding into all the small ischemic areas.

We need to get as many members of Christina's family here as possible,
Williams told the grief-stricken partner. We can't keep someone on life

support who has met the criteria for brain death. Finally, reluctantly, Anna agreed, and one by one Christina's family members surrounded her bed. Chase and Williams stood by as Anna sat on the bed and took Christina's hand in hers, one last time.

And suddenly, with a groan, Christina arched her back and squeezed, pulling Anna's hand to her. She continued arching her back, as though trying to sit up. Behind Williams and Chase, one of Christina's family let out a piercing scream. Both doctors knew immediately what was happening, although only Williams had seen it before. The phenomenon is called the Lazarus effect, or Lazarus syndrome, after the New Testament Lazarus who was raised from the dead by Jesus's touch. But this syndrome represented no restoration of life to the dead. It was purely a spinal reflex at work.

Just as the deep brain contains structures of clustered neurons – like those of the thalamus – the spinal cord has a series of nuclei or ganglia that ordinarily take commands from the brain to initiate loops of interconnected actions. The purpose of these spinal cord reflexes may be anything from snapping the body back from a roasting fire to leaping at an explosion. The knot of neurons powering a spinal reflex is not large—it might be all a roundworm gets for a brain—but it could drive a couple of very lifelike activities, and here before the onlookers were two. The seizing hand and arching spine represented one. The groan derived from nothing more than a reflex of the glottis, constricting the throat, and residual air forced out of the lungs by the arching of the spine. The phenomenon has been reported in morgues. Bodies awaiting embalming may actually sit up, straight from the prone, terrifying unprepared morgue workers out of their wits.

If she sits up, Chere said to herself, I go down. Please, God, do not let her sit up.

In a moment, as always, the reflex relaxed and Manning's dead form slumped backward onto the bed.

Williams, taking Anna's arm, explained to everyone what had happened. We took over for Christina's heart, he said, then gave her heroic levels of medications that would keep her blood pressure up even though her entire brain, brain stem included, stopped working many hours ago and is dead beyond any hope of reviving. Slowly, everyone quieted. Anna understood. The end had come. It was over. Chere prayed, Let that be that. But it was like praying before the call gods.

THE NEW UNIT WAS GORGEOUS. Six months ago, at the end of December, the barred doors beyond which chaos had reigned flew open to reveal half a makeover: more-spacious rooms, soft pastels of pink, green, tan, gray in two-tone in rooms and halls, colorful borders on the ceilings, posters to carry the reemerging imagination far, far away. After that, the "old" ICU had closed for the second round of reconstruction. Halsted 6 remained the backup unit, cramped and distant. In March, media day had welcomed Baltimore to the expanded Neuro Critical Care Unit of Johns Hopkins. At each end of the long hallways running from east to west on opposite sides of the central office block were nurses' stations, their edges beveled to offer clean lines and clear views. Dead center, between the two stations, was a physicians' office that in many ways was the highlight of the new "order." Here, after walking rounds ended each morning, everyone sat down for the lengthy and crucial nursing reports that wove the observations of the overnight shift into the plan for the day's treatment.

For Mirski, the nursing reports were the key to the unit's success, and nurses always opened walking rounds with observations of each of their two patients, though not necessarily at one time. First in order of business came patients who might be transferred to the floor that day, unless they were bumped in priority by patients in crisis. Then came the reports on each of as many as 22 patients in neuro critical care, in order of seriousness. These new sitdown rounds in the office might last two hours, consuming the bulk of the morning, but under Mirski's plan it was here that most of the former mess of paperwork was taken care of, where the transforming power of new technology showed itself.

A nurse walking in on sitdown rounds, usually standing in the doorway to report, saw as many as three of the doctors at computer terminals. To the far left would be the attending, entering into the hospital's Eclipsis system in one pass all the information needed to update patient status, log in drugs and other vital information and finally – a major boost in efficiency – entering all the information needed for billing, such as diagnostic codes and length of time spent in each category. Hit the ENTER key. Done.

At either of two laptops also hooked into the hospital's broadband, fellows and residents could update charts, call up CT or MRI scans or schedule them, and look up or alter the day's calendars. In many ways, the back and forth of the reports and questions masked the enormous electronic work going on as they all, individually and as a group, communicated their findings and questions to the hospital's computer-brain and retrieved the summations and calculated results.

To Mirski the importance of the efficient billing system could hardly be overstated. Most important, it provided more time for patient care, ever more in demand in the larger unit. But—no small consideration—it also reduced the challenges from insurance payers over the loss of documentation for claims for service. He had set out to prove the findings in Hawaii were no fluke, that managing neurointensive patients with experts would improve their outcomes and cut costs. Now he wanted to prove the unit would be a money maker for the hospital. With Bayview under its wing, the administration had accepted his plan to add a third two-year fellow to the team. That would mean that the professional skills of six physicians fully trained as neurologists, anesthesiologists or both, who now were becoming expert in neuro critical care, would be available in the unit.

He still chafed under the salary restrictions of the academic workplace. "The way the system is set up," Mirski often said, "at some point I will be forced to leave here. I have a family to be concerned about."

More seriously, just as Mirski was getting the new schedule under control, Anish Bhardwaj had gotten an offer that would be hard for him to refuse—not that Anish would be lured away by money. He had been offered the directorship of his own neurointensive care unit at a major university hospital in California. Mirski had assured Bhardwaj he would understand if he took it, though losing his intense service as deputy director would leave a huge hole in the division administration. Moving up was, after all, what they all trained and worked for. "The time is past when an academic clinician-investigator can just take care of patients and do research," Mirski explains. "At a point in your career you have to take a leadership role, and that means administration."

The lack of financial draw in academia was a fact of life. No one knew that better than Mirski, and he knew it limited the number of fellows who would follow through toward leadership of NICUs in teaching hospitals— though there were a fair number of teaching hospitals that were still for-profit, or at least did not operate under the stiff, break-even concept of academic institutions such as Johns Hopkins. He strongly suspected that Chere Chase would move toward private practice for that reason, though he would try to persuade her to stay on as junior faculty. Although he very much wanted Diana Greene-Chandos to complete her fellowship, he believed she would move away from the demands of academia, also for family reasons, though in her case more linked to quality family time than to financial needs.

B U T   T H A T   W A S   M U N D A N E   S T U F F. This brutal June week was not over by half, and here was another grim case. A young woman, 32, brain dead of a brain stem stroke, was a potential organ donor. Her family offered, feeling hopeful that some good could come of their loss. So Chase and Williams went through the long procedures of preparing for a "non-heartbeat donor," whose available organs would be taken in the operating room as soon as the final brain-death test was complete. On the brink. The lab tests come back in the middle of the night: hepatitis C positive. Organ donation was out.

Now came Jean Gall, brought in by EMTs on a 911 call by the man she lived with. She'd collapsed, apparently of a stroke. She'd had a stroke before. Boyfriend and parents were gathered. She was gone. Then one of neurology's stroke experts, came by with scans and noted that there was evidence of trauma as well as ischemic stroke. The family's ears perked up at that. Their eyes went to the boyfriend. And he admitted that, yes, they had been quarreling loudly right before her collapse, but, no, he had not struck her. The stroke expert said it was possible that medication had caused the swelling, instead of trauma. A case for the medical examiner.

Then an elderly mother of 13 was wheeled in dying, who had asked for "comfort measures only." She did not want to be revived but simply to be kept comfortable, since she was beyond cure. Twelve children and more family crowded around, one so upset he fainted and needed treatment for a leg injury from his fall. Finally child number 13 showed up and gasped, "You've got to save her! You've got to bring her back." And the others told Chase, "Let us take him outside, we'll change his mind."

"Absolutely not," Chase told them. "We're going to get together on this." And so they did, and the woman passed on peacefully.

Now came the capper, James Smith.

Smitty, marine veteran who never quite made it home from the war. A drifter who would show up at his mother's house from time to time, hang around, often silently. Sometimes drunk, sometimes just out of it. A long history of alcohol and who knows what. He had showed up again, no money in his pocket, a huge abrasion on his forehead. Alcohol again, his mother said, taking him in. He'd often had seizures from alcohol withdrawal, may have had one or more right then. There he sat on the couch staring, not moving, as he had done so often before. But this time, after 12 hours, he slumped over. His mother called 911.

Smitty had had a massive subdural hemorrhage. Subdural meaning it had occurred in the space between the outermost and toughest of the brain's three membrane layers and the fine, delicate inner two. That was serious enough, but the huge pooling blood pocket quickly throttled his brain to death. He arrived brain dead. And then came the twilight zone.

Williams and Chase took Mary Smith aside and Williams explained in his ever gentle way that there was nothing they could do for James. He was going to die.

And Mary replied, "What are his chances?"

Pause.

He really doesn't have any chances, Williams explained. The pressure inside his brain has robbed it of oxygen for so long he cannot recover.

How long will it be, Mary asked, until you can take him off that machine?

Soon Mary Smith's goddaughter arrived, not a moment too soon. They had wondered if Mary might be suffering from dementia, though her grief for her "injured" son was enormous and who knew what grief might do.

The goddaughter, Janice, whom Chase remembers as intensely religious in her conversation, told them her own mother had just died. Mary had been so much like a mother to Janice, though – as her mother had been to James—that Janice was forgoing her own mother's wake to be at Mary's side. She quoted prolifically from the Bible to Mary, who prayed over James.

Mary seemed to be one of those "concrete" people, who needed to see in order to understand, to hold on to a visceral sense of reality. At least that was how it seemed to the physicians trying to navigate toward an unavoidable end. So Williams decided, for the first time in the history of the unit, to allow Mary and Janice to be present for the final series of brain death tests, in which they would "walk" down the brain stem by testing first higher-level then, descending step by step, lower-level brain stem reflexes. Across town, Maryland Shock Trauma, like some other U.S. hospitals, was routinely allowing families to be present for end-of-life measures in the belief that that helped bring closure.

This final procedure would end, of course, with the apnea test. If there was no gasp for breath from the lowest brain stem as James's brain cells choked on carbon dioxide, he was dead. That gasp is the most primitive of all reflexes in the lower brain stem.

But, Janice said, there was still another, truer way of knowing if James was dead or not. After they've finished the tests, she told Mary, if James is still not breathing, you must do this: at the very top of your voice, scream out three times, "Lazarus, come forth!" Chase's heart all but stopped. *Please, God, no.*

In a short rite that preceded the final test, they read a note a friend had left on James's bed. "Hey, Smitty, here to see you. Don't die. You were always here for me. Sorry I couldn't be here for you."

Williams began the apnea test. "You can put your hand on his chest," he consoled Mary, and she did. "He's breathing!" she cried out. "My baby's breathing."

Yes, Williams explained, that's because the machine is breathing for him. He is not responding. I'm so sorry.

CO_2 normalized. Chase's heart is pounding in her chest. James's heart is pounding in his, pumped full of pressors. Now Williams turns the respirator off.

"Now!" Janice cries out. "You have to yell out now. 'Lazarus, come forth!'"

But Mary, quiet, cannot bring out a shout, instead says quietly, "Don't leave me, baby. Come on, come back." She moans that she has lost five children this year. "Come back," she says.

"Now!" Janice says. "Yell, 'Lazarus, come forth!'"

No breathing. Chase watches the monitor. The heart is going through last, agonal beats. In moments it will stop. Blood pressure, which had been sky high from the pressors, is drifting down like a leaf.

Now there is one last step, the gesture to ease the suddenness of loss. "We're going to turn the respirator back on again," Williams says, describing the steps of the protocol.

"What? No!" Janice barked. "He's dead. Don't you dare do that."

Williams halted in midstep. "No?"

"He's dead," she repeated. Then, wearily, "We know he's dead now."

And that *was that*, at least for them.

The patient's nurse always faces the real last step, usually alone. Smitty was the first patient his young nurse had ever lost, so Chase stayed with her to share the task. Tagging the big toe for the morgue. Encasing the dead patient in a body bag. Turning out the light.

MORNING ON MEYER 7. "I'm glad you're here, doctor," the first patient says, so clearly you wonder why he's in the hospital at all. "Thanks for coming over." He thinks the white-coated team is visiting him at home. He is partially paralyzed from a stroke on his left side, and they are trying to determine which of his perceptions might be dimmed. So the tests begin: "Can you find your left ear with your right hand?" He moves straight and true in the correct direction, but misses. He plainly cannot feel his own presence on that side. Another test question: "Look right at me and tell me which finger I'm touching." The correct answer brings a few smiles: "My flip-off finger."

Time for sit-down rounds. Betsy Zink comes into the doorway of the physicians' room. Her patient this morning is set for aspirin and the blood thinner and clot fighter Coumadin. Like Okoye and Takahashi, Zink is a Nurse Clinician III. She heads a group of five other nurses and serves on the code committee, charged with maintaining unit competency in advanced life-support techniques. Zink also teaches a range of classes for new nurses. And, like all the others, she schedules her own shifts within the framework of staffing needs while she works on a master of science in critical care and trauma nursing.

To surpass the "expert level" of II, Zink had to prove she could supervise the entire nursing staff and run the unit in Ski Lower's absence. She has to able to carry out the duties of all other nursing positions, like those of the charge nurse who schedules beds and juggles assignments according to the numbers of patients, illnesses, vacations; or the jobs of the techs who do EKGs, administer IVs, draw blood.

But now she is asked to recall a patient of a few hundred mornings ago. Does she remember Jay Lokeman? "Sure. He was the nicest guy in the unit," she says. Her regular 12-hour shift had ended at 7 p.m. that Saturday, before Lokeman's crisis, but she was there through subsequent bouts with kidney and other problems, when it seemed he would die or be left a living wreck. But he recovered, and she remembers him well in the days and weeks afterward. Affable, good-humored. "Everybody liked him—nurses, patients, doctors."

HE SITS IN HIS SISTER Cathy Reid's house in Columbia, elbows on knees, smiles, thinks about his past, worries over the future. He is visiting her for the weekend. This afternoon they had taken Cathy's 7-year-old niece to see *The Two Towers* and had just gotten home. Jay is now living in a halfway house in downtown Baltimore. Soon he hopes to move to less-regimented quarters, but he has chosen this for himself. He's been clean six months and wants to make that forever. He frequently goes to meetings of Narcotics Anonymous, regularly visits a counselor.

He skewers his problem with the ease with which one might describe a lifelong enemy. "Everyone around me is a superstar," Jay says. "And that's just how it was. I just wasn't very good in school. I didn't have any self-esteem." So when he was finally clean, each time, it was that that got him down. He often struggled through the craving period successfully, as though cured—right before Johns Hopkins it had been a whole year.

And after leaving Johns Hopkins that summer, he was winning the struggle again. He'd planned to go back to work for the same collection agency he had been working for as an account manager. But he looked at himself, where he was at 33, and he hated what he saw. It was the failure in the mirror who went back to the coke and, sometimes, heroin. For a while on the coke he liked himself. Everything was okay.

Then the ripping and running would begin. Paranoia would creep in. People would be after him. He would take off in terror, in any weather, in the middle of the night or broad daylight. And as for being hit by the car, the accident that had put him in Maryland General, that was par for the course. Years earlier he had hobbled home from

Georgia on crutches, with two broken ankles, telling Cathy he'd been in a car accident. "Actually, I was some place I had absolutely no business being," he says flatly. "I was thrown right out of a fourth story window." He shakes his head, looks over with that *Can you believe that?* expression people get when they don't know what to make of someone's bizarre behavior.

Then there was that afternoon in mid-July, arms still aching from the pins holding him together, back on the coke again, and the world closing in. All he can remember is running at top speed, more than a mile, from his apartment on the North Side down to the condo where his father lived, seeking refuge. What he would like now and would look for was a job working with people. He loves working with people, and except for his job as a tennis coach years ago, his jobs have always isolated him from other people.

On the other hand, he knows this is all up to him alone. His family loves him, but he has to do this by himself. So he will give it his best.

How about taking a picture of him?

Okay.

With Cathy?

No, no. Just by myself.

No supports. A good-looking young guy in slacks and sweater looks up into the camera. He sits with arms wrapped around crossed legs, before a crackling fire, his smile easy and confident.

Tentative victory. As with Jack Apple, Gail Beck and all the others, you hold onto such good moments and want to fit them into a pattern. You want to see a promising pattern being established in a smooth curve on the chart. But the curve is erratic and there may be no pattern. The victory is tentative now; it may be solid tomorrow.

A PHONE CALL to Warrenton, Virginia. Sharon Arent? *Speaking.*
How is Chad?

After the shunt at Johns Hopkins, she says Chad began improving
steadily from the quiet, absent figure last seen that early July. The shunt revision was a blessing. She is certain that "the old Chad's still there." The
family returns to Johns Hopkins regularly for tests to make sure the shunt
remains working. Mike Williams has become Chad's neurologist and is very
impressed with his response to neuro tests, as he shows in his reports.

Chad plainly enjoys being wheeled onto their deck when it snows,
turning his face up to feel the flakes. And a sure-fire indication of his return: once again he hates tomatoes. He responds to questions, though
slowly and with babyish vocalization, but still distinct. *Uh-huh, un-unh* at
the right times. And spontaneously: *Thank you.* Or out of the blue: *Love you.*

Sharon Arent remains as convinced as she was in the worst hours after Chad's rollover accident: "I truly believe that one day he will be living
independently. Maybe not in his own apartment, but with minor assis-
tance. Talking, independent."

Mike Williams cannot confirm all that the Arents believe, he says. But
he quickly adds that he doesn't doubt any of it. There is only so much
tests and numbers can show, only so much even a neurointensivist can glean
from hard data.

THE LAST DAY OF JUNE opens a new week as it closes the academic year. The incoming fellows are already on board, being fitted for
coats, briefed on hospital procedure, prepped for their grueling residents'
call. Another photo will be hung on the wall. It is Diana Greene-Chandos's
last day in the unit. She would have preferred to finish the fellowship, she
says, but not at the cost to family she saw it running up. She has found a
job that will put her into both the neuro critical care world and the more

scheduled life of a private practitioner. She is joining a group of neurologists contracted with Howard County Hospital to provide the range of neuro services that might be needed—including critical care. That will be her role as the group's director of critical care neurology. She will still be a hospitalist in many ways, and still in the orbit of Johns Hopkins, which owns Howard County Hospital. And she and Brandon plan to have more children. Indeed, in the fall she will tell Chere she is expecting the following August.

Anish Bhardwaj, to everyone's joy and relief, has decided to remain as codirector in the unit. To persuade him to give up the chance to run his own NICU in California, the administration named him vice chairman of Neurology, an appointment Mirski says will bode well for Bhardwaj's chances of getting a top chairmanship one day.

ROOM 731, where Rita Serianni, Donna Soja, and Jennie Ray had each spent hard first nights in the unit, still gets the tough cases, given that it's at the "most intensive" end of the unit, the room nearest the electric double doors. Diana Greene-Chandos had watched with deep concern as Jennie's Glasgow Coma Scale score had plunged from near-normal 13 to barely in the world at 6, rise again, and fall. A bad sign. But those who recover can only recover memories that were laid down to begin with, so their recollections of their days in the NICU, like Jack Apple's, are stitched together out of high-conscious hours and days.

"I really wasn't that sick," Jennie says, even now, back on campus at Vassar on a blustery Saturday afternoon. "They thought I had a seizure at first, but I don't think I ever did, and I haven't had any since."

She does remember the "left field cut" in her vision from the AVM, because she still has it. She has seen Greg Bergey, Johns Hopkins chief epileptologist, and he says her vision may return to normal. But the field cut is little more than an annoyance, she says. "I'm not even aware of it, unless someone talks to me and I realize I should be seeing them from where they're standing, but I have to turn my head a little." She had to practice driving again, to make sure she turned her head enough to catch cars in the missing field area.

The AVM is gone. In December, just before returning to Vassar for the second half of her senior year, she had gone to Neuroradiology, and Rafael Tamargo and Kieran Murphy had fused the small, clustered web of misformed artery-vein connections, so her blood now flowed normally through other nearby vessels. Not all AVMs are cured so simply, since some involve critical blood vessels.

She had spent fall semester at home, carrying out her assignments, writing papers and short stories, and conversing with her professors over the Internet. Now she was about to plunge into her senior thesis, due in a couple of months. It would be a collection of short stories—a creative thesis, as her mother had said she would write. Today, though, was a celebration.

Her parents, Jack and Nancy, had driven up, because tonight she would sing with the Madrigal Singers in a great old restored theater in downtown Poughkeepsie, New York. They would perform Aaron Copeland's *In the Beginning*. A soprano, she had also resumed singing with the campus opera group.

Reminded how sure she was that Jennie would be here, doing just these things, Nancy smiled. "I really believed it would turn out. I just believed it would."

Once More . . .

*How does the brain work, and how do you protect
the brain? A problem getting worse instead of better
as the population ages. Tackling big, difficult
problems like that, that's our strength.*

EDWARD MILLER, M.D.
President and Chief Executive Officer
Johns Hopkins Medicine
July

I T ' S C A L L E D the NICU's "Daily
Template":

"6:00–7:30 a.m. Prerounds.
Participants: All residents, both fellows, attending neurointensivist, night/day nurses. Nurse
reports: Major events overnight, changes in neurological exam, vitals summary, and any other issues that need M.D. attention or would affect transfer potential . . . "

Rounds begin an hour earlier every day in what Marek Mirski is sure comprises "the largest, closed neurointensive care unit in the world." *Closed* is still the key word. Neurointensive specialists alone manage all 22 patients in the beds stretching along the corridors on either side of Meyer 7, plus those in the eight beds of Bayview's NICU. The specialized neurointensive nurses, ranking from Nurse Clinician I to III, care for all of them, two patients per nurse per shift.

Mirski does not hedge on the importance of the nurses to the expansion of the unit: it could not have been carried out without their being empowered, he says. His problem, he knew, would be to spread a constant number of physicians over a vastly increased patient population while assuring that there would be no drop in care. That meant more responsibility for the nurses. The addition of the third fellow would mean one more junior and one more senior fellow in the two-year pool. But the number of residents available was fixed, because their training was supported by federal money. And the residents, with their long call schedules, provided the heaviest coverage in the unit. His response was to triage the NICU.

At the east end of the NICU is the "most intensive" nursing station, at the west end the station for "neurovascular critical care"—postoperative patients and others who are relatively stable. All get the same nursing coverage, while the fellows and residents concentrate their attention on the most critical patients, just yards away.

Though he may disdain the military model of medical training for its inflexibility and harshness, Mirski has created, of necessity, a model of rounds that looks much like a military drill. While prerounds move along from 6 to 7:30 a.m., the attending or fellow assigned to triage is carrying out that work for the day, and the fellow assigned to the neurosurgery team is on those rounds from 7 to 7:30 a.m. From 7:30 to 7:50, X-ray rounds for all physicians on the team, who then move on to discuss the unit's sickest patients with their nurses until 8:15. The junior fellow and the charge nurse then quickly come up with the order in which patients will be discussed in "work rounds," the new, sit-down rounds that will run until 11 a.m.

That leaves the rest of the day "free" — for procedures, orders carried out, lectures, administration, emergencies, consults, studies. At least until 4:30, when evening walking rounds begin. They will run until 6 p.m., but it is not unusual for them to stretch an hour longer.

"The system works," Mirski says. It must. He expects a 50 percent increase in neurosurgery patients over the next few years and more stroke patients in the NICU.

Far from incapacitating the attending physicians for their research, their out-of-unit time continues to be among the most productive in the hospital, he says. Mirski's own salary is covered 20 percent by grant support, and others even more so. "Romer Geocadin, Michel Torbey, Anish Bhardwaj, they're all heavily funded" by NIH grants, Mirski says, and he believes the division has more such external funding than any other in the hospital. "Some members of our faculty are so well funded that they could cover their salaries without even working in the Neuro Intensive Care Unit."

Among the recent publications, a book chapter out of the work in Dave Sherman's lab: "Mirski M.A., Sherman D.L., Ziai W.C. Stimulation for Epilepsy: Anterior thalamus and the Pentylenetetrazol Model." In: Luders, H. (Ed.), *Brain Stimulation and Epilepsy,* Cleveland Clinic, Cleveland, 2002.

Mirski's future? "It's pretty obvious I've been grooming myself for some kind of senior level administrative position," he says. Over time, that might mean giving up the operating room, and his research would have to taper off. He likes research — the opportunity to plunge more deeply into his own epilepsy investigations and take part in clinical trials helped bring him back from Hawaii. But if he had to make a choice between giving all his time to research or to the clinic, it would be easy. "I would take the clinic. I'm a good investigator, I think, but a better clinician." And sometimes there is the lure of the "small-town doctor," which Hawaii offered in some ways, that place where everyone knows you. Still, he finds the atmosphere among all the units involved in neuroscience at Johns Hopkins collegial enough to make up for that.

Whatever Mirski's plans for the unit, they seem in sync with the larger world of Johns Hopkins. We sit in the office of Edward L. Miller, not long ago the head of anesthesiology, now the CEO of the whole shebang.

In part, Miller sounds like the CEO of any Fortune 500 company with a high-end product and a highly skilled work force: "We don't want to be in the commodities business," he says. "There's been too much invested in this faculty to do the routine. Our goal has always been to push the frontier forward." On the other hand, this is a nonprofit: "Johns Hopkins strives to be a break-even institution. We simply cannot run in the red."

The fact is that Miller is CEO of a $2.5 billion operation, counting the hospital and health system, medical school, and all the affiliates from Bayview and Howard County medical centers to Johns Hopkins/Singapore. And that operation exists to discover answers to new problems and to unsolved age-old problems — which could be a definition of research. Yes, Johns Hopkins will remain a top hospital for patients, he says. But its survival depends on garnering research dollars from the NIH and private philanthropy. His job is leverage — to balance the currently highly profitable medical school, home base for research, against the barely profitable hospital; that could change, he says, as it has in the past. In that case he'll reverse the leverage.

But the core will always be research, discovery. "Take a look at one of the great unsolved problems: How does the brain work? And how do you protect the brain?" Given all the things medicine can do well, Miller says, "if you don't have a brain that works, there is not much sense in the rest." He adds, "What Marek and others have done is to concentrate the resources on these big problems, and that's what we do best."

I SWORE I WOULD END the story here, with the summer of 2002 drawing to a close, everything tidy. Mirski and I decided we would have coffee on this quiet Saturday, a slow day in the unit. And never again would I allow the real world to intrude on my wrapping up the story by updating it — that is, by altering my recorded history. Reality would not, in that nasty way it has, slip a tentacle from the present backward into the past, distorting what I was setting down before the ink dried. This story would have been different if I had stuck to that resolve.

For example, at that "closing" moment, I had never spoken with Jay Lokeman himself, in the flesh. His mother, sister, brother had all spoken openly, in hopes Jay would see all he meant to them. Then one day my cell phone rang, and it was Cathy Reid. Her brother was on the phone and wanted to talk to me. Away I went, like a leaf in a wind tunnel.

And as the summer of 2002 closes, Tammy Brasher is still alive, struggling bravely to hang on, and I have not yet tracked down Joe Rose and learned the truth. There's more, of course. Imagine that in September, 2002, I had suddenly found the science of predicting the future. Looking confidently forward I could say: in late April, 2003, Jennie Ray will have three grand mal seizures in a row, the first she's ever had, in the apartment she shares with a friend while working at a private school in Baltimore. Three weeks later, she will get a phone call from me and talk about it all as cheerfully as ever, and as full of wry, self-deprecating humor.

There is a 100 percent chance that as June rolls around again, Chere Chase will immediately take on direction of her own unit. Forsyth Medical Center in Winston-Salem, North Carolina, will hire her as director of Stroke and Cerebrovascular Medicine, and her first order of business will be to create an acute stroke care program. She also will set up an education program to assure that EMTs and other health care professionals recognize the first signs of stroke and to assure that everyone moves patients through the hospital system during their early "golden hours" for treatment and recovery.

BUT I'VE JUMPED AHEAD. We are still back in the present late summer 2002, looking forward to that final coffee. As for that and Mirski's quiet Saturday, you would think he had danced before the call gods. To hear him tell it, though, this might have been just another day at the office. Chere Chase is now a seasoned, senior neurointensivist fellow, otherwise, the weekend could not unfold as it does. Mirski, wrapping up his turn as attending in the NICU, is also finishing out two days as neuroanesthesiologist, the kind of schedule almost no one else would keep.

On Friday, a neuro trauma had reached the emergency room in the usual scream of sirens and rush of paramedics wheeling a gurney to the waiting trauma team. Bill Damino, only 17 years old, was shooting hoops with friends when he dropped like a stone. Confirmed: an aneurysm, which may have bled but did not ruptured.

Mirski had not planned on doing any neuroanesthesia Saturday. But he knew the chief anesthesia resident was on call this weekend, as was the chief neurosurgery resident. That meant the OR was pretty well covered in support, so he saw no problem in taking this case himself. Things looked good for neurosurgery for the Damino boy, first thing tomorrow. Neal Naff, last noted as Dan Hanley's partner in IVH trials, was the neurosurgeon on call. So Mirski signed Damino onto the Saturday schedule, with himself as neuroanesthesiologist. He would carry rounds in the NICU in the morning, but Chase would be comfortable taking over afterward. She could write notes, and everyone would know where to find him.

Saturday. Round they go, clicking along in the new daily drill. Half an hour into rounds came the code alarm. The whoop-whoop-whoop, as riveting as an air raid siren, alerted that a patient right here in the Neuro ICU was coding, going into cardiac arrest. They rushed into Carl James's room to find Obi Okoye working over him. Mirski saw from the monitor that James had not in fact coded—yet. Okoye had been running through the neuro exam and realized from James's responses and her long experience that he was crashing. James was Alex Olivi's patient; he had just had an aneurysm clipped, and the scans showed no signs of any other aneurysms, or any other brain abnormality.

"Let's get him breathing here." Mirski manages to get a tongue depressor part way in before it snaps in half, but that's enough space to force an air tube. Sure enough, the monitor shows respiration settling well at that moment. But look at the patient: no response to voice, eyes wide and staring straight ahead. Frozen.

Time for a CT. While that's going on, Mirski heads to the OR to find everything going smoothly, the difficult part of Damino's surgery still hours away, the team just prepping the room. But on his way back up, he learns both of James's pupils are blown. He looks dead.

The resident has Alex Olivi on the line, telling him his patient is in crisis. Mirski takes the phone. "In my estimation," Mirski tells him, "this is an aneurysm that needs attention emergently."

"I'm on my way," Olivi says.

Soon the CTs confirm that the aneurysm is a new one that hadn't shown up, and it bled. It is not the one Olivi already clipped.

Keeping score: this means Mirski will have two simultaenous cases as neuroanesthesiologist — not unusual, except both are weekend emergencies involving aneurysms, both of which have bled.

James's case is scheduled for an OR way down the hall from Damino's. That will never work. Mirski talks the scheduling nurse into moving James to the largest OR on the floor, which is right next to the Damino boy's. Olivi will soon be scrubbing in. Naff is back to work on Damino.

A small window of time opens. Mirski scrubs out, heads up to the Neuro ICU, and meets with the wife and sister of another critical patient to discuss issues that had emerged on new scans. Five minutes later, his pager sends him two quick messages that say, Come now.

At the OR doors to scrub in, a nurse comes out to tell him Damino's bleeding aneurysm now has ruptured. Very serious, but not a catastrophe, not when Damino is now in midsurgery, under scope, with neurosurgeon Naff right there. With the chief anesthesia resident in charge, Mirski needs only to make sure the right protocol is being followed. Soon Naff would have a temporary clip on the aneurysm, buying time.

No such luck. The aneurysm had ruptured as Naff was placing the temporary clip, and instead of a penny-size circle of blood, the intraoperative monitor screen showed nothing but blood. Maybe a bit of carotid artery there, or optic nerve, but it was all vanishing under a red pool.

"Dr. Mirski," a voice at his side says, "you're wanted next door."

"What is it?"

"Mr. James's aneurysm has ruptured."

Oh, sweet . . . Two ruptured aneurysms.

Mirski ducks next door and there is Olivi with his gloved finger in the dike – or at least, literally, on it. Blood is filling the bucket, and they order up replacements. "Actually we're okay here," Mirski tells Olivi, "because we're transfusing him as fast as he's bleeding. By the time you need more blood, it'll be here, and I'll be back."

Next door they are still suctioning and probing the Damino boy's bleeding incision, and the resident on that case, too, is ordering up more blood. Good. This bleeding doesn't look too bad. That's when Mirski notices that one of the nurses has his hand under the drapes.

"What's he doing?" Mirski asks.

"He's got his finger on the carotid, to stem the surging blood."

Not good.

"Would you benefit from having a clean field?" Mirski asks Naff.

Yes, he answers.

"Let me turn the pressure extremely low," Mirski says. "You won't have much time. Put a clip on the carotid, maybe two."

Done.

Three minutes later: "I'm going to bring the pressure back up."

"Why?" But a rhetorical question. Naff knew very well why.

"I don't want him to die," Mirski said. Damino's brain had been without new blood for most of three minutes.

"Do what you have to do," Neff says.

It works. The clip is on. He slowly begins relieving the carotid clip, pressure of blood surging back into the brain mounting gradually. The clip holds. The aneurysm is sealed. One down. Exit Mirski.

Enter Mirski. Just in time to see Olivi testing the aneurysm clip with his gloved finger. As complicated a bubble of artery as you could find, this one trifurcated, ballooned into three bulbs.

The riskiest piece of neurosurgery, aneurysm clipping, here multiplied by two. Done under emergency conditions. Mirski heads down to angio a few hours later, where Kieran Murphy's scans shows that both patients' clips are neatly seated.

The end: Damino and James are wheeled into the NICU within three minutes of each other. Mirski joins Chase to talk to the families.

So much for that. So much for coffee. So much for a quiet Saturday.

Rounds and call finished and the electronic "paperwork" of the unit under control, Mirski takes off in his old Subaru wagon for the car dealership. He traded in his Toyota two-seater for this Subaru when Kara was born, 13 years ago. For weeks he's had his eye on a new sports car, a hardtop that's one of the few that will hold four people comfortably. It isn't just for him. Kara will be driving in a few years, followed in two by Erin. It's a beauty. He takes it out for a spin and drives it home that day.

Index

OTHER DANA PRESS BOOKS AND PERIODICALS

THE BARD ON THE BRAIN Understanding the Mind Through the Art of Shakespeare and the Science of Brain Imaging, Paul Matthews, M.D. and Jeffrey McQuain. Foreword by Diane Ackerman.
Exploring the beauty and mystery of the human mind and the workings of the brain, following the path Bard pointed out in 35 of the most famous speeches from his plays. 100 color illustrations. 248 pp. 9 x 9.

0-9723830-2-6 $35.00

STRIKING BACK AT STROKE A Doctor-Patient Journal, Cleo Hutton, and Louis R. Caplan, M.D.
A personal account with medical guidance for anyone enduring the changes that a stroke can bring to a life, a family, and a sense of self. 15 illustrations. 240 pp. 6x9

0-9723830-1-8 $27.00

THE DANA GUIDE TO BRAIN HEALTH, Floyd E. Bloom, M.D., M. Flint Beal, M.D. and David J. Kupfer, M.D., Editors. Foreword by William Safire.
A home reference on the brain edited by three leading experts collaborating with 104 distinguished scientists and medical professionals. In lay language with cross references and advice on 72 conditions such as autism and Alzheimer's disease to multiple sclerosis, depression, and Parkinson's disease. Sixteen-page color section; 200 black and white illustrations. 768 pp. 7¼ x 9¼ (Published by The Free Press)

0-7492-0397 $45.00

UNDERSTANDING DEPRESSION What We Know and What You Can Do About It, J. Raymond DePaulo Jr., M.D. and Leslie Alan Horvitz. Foreword by Kay Redfield Jamison.
What depression is, who gets it and why, what happens in the brain, troubles that come with the illness, and the treatments that work. 304 pp. 9½ x 6½ (Co-published with John Wiley & Sons, Inc.)

0-471-39552-8 $24.95

KEEP YOUR BRAIN YOUNG The Complete Guide to Physical and Emotional Health and Longevity, Guy Mc Khann, M.D. and Marilyn Albert, Ph.D.
Every aspect of aging and the brain: changes in memory, nutrition, mood, sleep, and sex, as well as the later problems in alcohol use, vision, hearing, movement and balance. 304 pp. 6⅛ x 9¼ (Co-published with John Wiley & Sons, Inc.)

0-471-43028-5 $15.95

THE END OF STRESS AS WE KNOW IT, Bruce McEwen, Ph.D. with Elizabeth Norton Lasley. Foreword by Robert Sapolsky.
How brain and body work under stress and how it is possible to avoid its debilitating effects. 239 pp. 6 x 9 (Co-published with Joseph Henry Press)

0-309-07640-4 $27.95

A GOOD START AT LIFE: Understanding Your Child's Brain and Behavior, Norbert Herschkowitz, M.D. and Elimore Chapman Herschkowitz, M.A.
Development from prenatal to age 6, with particular attention to how social competency and personality unfold. Each chapter includes a question and answer section on everyday issues in child development. Nine black and white illustrations; 4 stages-of-development charts. 283 pp. 6 x 9 (Co-published with Joseph Henry Press)

0-309-07639-0 $22.95

IN SEARCH OF THE LOST CORD: Solving the Mystery of Spinal Cord Regeneration written by award-winning popular medical writer Luba Vikhanski.
The story of the scientists and science involved in the international scientific race to find ways to repair the damaged spinal cord and restore movement. Twenty-one black and white photos; 12 illustrations. 269 pp. 6 x 9. (Co-published with Joseph Henry Press)

0-309-07437-1 $27.95

THE SECRET LIFE OF THE BRAIN, by Richard Restak, foreword by David Grubin.
Companion book to the PBS series of the same name, exploring recent discoveries about the brain from infancy through old age. Color photos and illustrations throughout. 201 pp. 8 x 10. (Co-published with Joseph Henry Press)

0-309-07435-5 $35.00

THE LONGEVITY STRATEGY How to Live to 100 Using the Brain-Body Connection, David Mahoney and Richard Restak, M.D. Foreword by William Safire. Advice on the brain and aging well. 272 pp. 5½ x 8½. (Co-published with John Wiley & Sons, Inc)

0-471-32794-8 $14.95

STATES OF MIND New Discoveries about How Our Brains Make Us Who We Are, Roberta Conlan, Editor.
Adapted from the Dana/Smithonian Associates lecture series by eight of the country's top brain scientists, including the 2000 Nobel laureate in medicine, Eric Kandel. 224 pp. 5½ x 8½. (Co-published with John Wiley & Sons, Inc.)

0-471-39973-6 $18.95

NEUROETHICS: Mapping the Field Conference Proceedings, Steven J. Marcus, Editor. Proceedings of the landmark 2002 conference organized by Stanford University and the University of California, San Francisco, at which more than 150 neuroscientists, bioethics, psychiatrists and psychologists, philosophers, and professors of law and public policy debated the implications of neuroscience research findings for individual and societal decision making. Photos and illustrations, 367 pp. 6 x 9.

0-972-3830-X

THE DANA SOURCEBOOK OF BRAIN SCIENCE: Resources for Secondary and Post-Secondary Teachers and Students.
A basic introduction to brain science, its history, current understanding of the brain, new developments, and future directions. Color and black and white photos; line illustrations. 164 pp., 8½ x 11.

ACTS OF ACHIEVEMENT The Role of Performing Arts Centers in Education.
Profiles of 60+ programs, eight extended case studies, from urban and rural communities across the United States, illustrating different approaches to performing arts-education programs in school settings. 164 pp. 8½ x 11.

PLANNING AN ARTS-CENTERED SCHOOL: A Handbook.
A practical guide for those interested in creating, maintaining, or upgrading arts-centered schools. Includes curriculum and development, governance, funding, assessment, and community participation. 164 pp., 3 color illustrations, 10 black and white illustrations. 8½ x 11.

PERIODICALS

CEREBRUM:The Dana Forum on Brain Science
A quarterly journal for general readers with feature articles, debates, and book reviews dealing with the latest discoveries about the brain and their implications for individuals and society.

Subscription (4 issues): $30/year ($42 foreign; $48 institutions)
To order a trial copy: call 1-877-860-0901 or write to Cerebrum Subscriber Services,
P.O. Box 573, Oxon Hill, MD 20745-0573

BRAINWORK: The Neuroscience Newsletter
A bimonthly, full color, 8-page newsletter for general readers reporting the latest findings in brain research.

Free: order through or download from www.dana.org/press

THE BRAIN IN THE NEWS
A monthly 8-page newspaper reprinting news and feature articles about brain research from leading newspapers and magazines in the U.S and abroad during the previous month.

Free: by mail only; order through www.dana.org/press

IMMUNOLOGY IN THE NEWS
A quarterly 8-page newspaper reprinting news and feature articles about immune system research, disease treatment and prevention, and biodefense from U.S. and foreign newspapers and scientific journals.

Free: by mail only; order through www.dana.org/press

ARTS EDUCATION IN THE NEWS
A quarterly 8-page newspaper reprinting news and feature articles about performing arts education in the schools from leading U.S. newspapers and magazines.

Free: by mail only; order through www.dana.org/press

VISIONS OF THE BRAIN: A Progress Report on Brain Research.
Published in March annually since 1995, the Progress Report, a publication of the Dana Alliance for Brain Initiatives, identifies the most significant findings from the previous year in brain research .

Free: order through or download from www.dana.org/press

BRAIN CONNECTIONS: Your Source Guide to Information on Brain Disease and Disorders.
Pocket-size 48-page booklet listing more than 275 organizations that help people with a brain related disorder and those responsible for their care and treatment. A publication of the Dana Alliance for Brain Initiatives. Listings include toll-free numbers, web-site and email addresses and regular mailing addresses.

Free: order through or download from www.dana.org